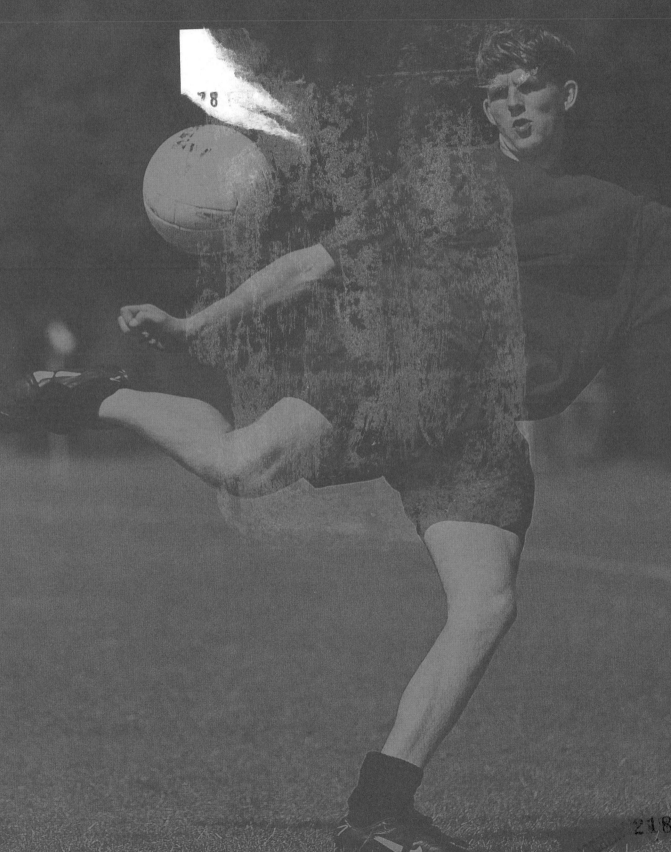

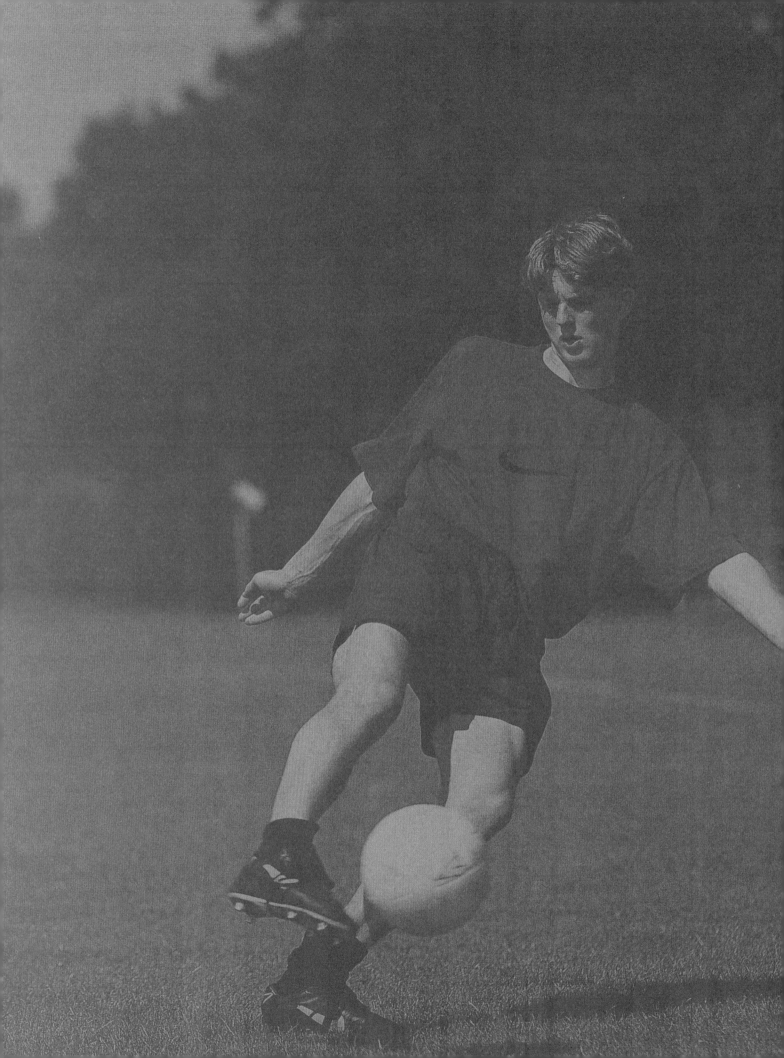

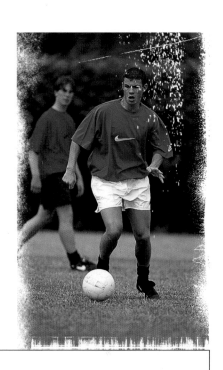

FOOTBALL FITNESS&SKILLS

PETE EDWARDS

HAMLYN

SPECIALLY COMMISSIONED
PHOTOGRAPHY BY ACTION PLUS

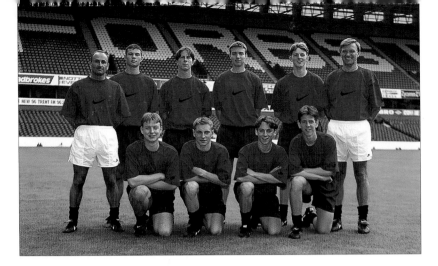

author's note

There are many people to thank for their hard work on this book. Firstly, I would like to thank Dave Smith for helping to put my ideas into words so skilfully. I am also grateful to Mick Raynor and Steve Beaglehole for their advice and assistance on the technique and tactics sections. Finally, I should like to thank the many people who worked so hard on the photographic shoot at Nottingham Forest's training ground: Richard Francis (the ever patient photographer), Mick Raynor (particularly for sacrificing a Saturday morning!), the Nottingham Forest youth team (whose good humour and good skill kept us smiling for the whole three days) and Jim Pearson and Julie at Nike (for providing the players' kits and my own!).

editor's note

This project would not have been possible without the hard work, patience and good humour of writer and sometime midfield dynamo Dave Smith. With any luck Dave will return to Sunday League football none the worse for his experience on this project – his football is bound to have improved, though I'm not so sure about his emotional stability. Maximal thanks Smudge.

dedication

I would like to dedicate this book to my wife Mair and children Siân, Daniel and Bryn. Thank you for all your support and encouragement.

acknowledgements

Publishing Director: Laura Bamford
Editor: Adam Ward
Art Director: Keith Martin
Design Manager: Bryan Dunn
Design: Martin Topping
Picture research: Jenny Faithful and Maria Gibbs
Commissioned photography: Richard Francis (Action Plus)
Kit and footwear: Nike UK

First published in Great Britain in 1997 by Hamlyn, an imprint of Reed Consumer Books Limited, Michelin House, 81 Fulham Road, London SW3 6RB and Auckland, Melbourne, Singapore and Toronto

Copyright © Hamlyn Limited 1997

ISBN 0 600 59132 8

Produced by Mandarin Offset
Printed in China

fitness 6

developing your technique 72

tactics 112

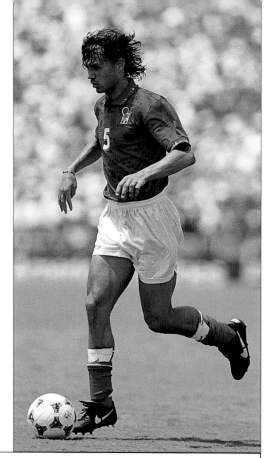

Paolo Maldini is not only one of the most skilful players in the world, he is also one of the fittest. To be successful in football, you must combine technical ability with hard work.

'With the right preparation and application, all footballers will improve their performances and get more from their football.'

introduction

The above is the honest and confident belief of fitness expert Pete Edwards, the brains behind this book and the man whose training ideals are attracting a great deal of attention in England.

His methods, outlined in full over the next 124 pages, are different and we all know that the problem with the British is that they are averse to change. But most now realise that the time has come to move on and mix the best of British with the best from the continent.

The popular belief that many European nations – the Italians in particular – are technically and physically superior is challenged by Pete Edwards, who believes all players can compete equally. And that's where this book comes in. The guidelines and suggestions set out will be new and exciting to some, revolutionary and frightening to others.

The Euro 96 anthem of 'Football's Coming Home' could be re-written to read 'Football's Moving On'. The question is: do you want to move on with it – or do you want to be left behind? If the former, the answer is simple; it is contained in this book.

'Look after yourself and your talent will look after you' is a statement which Pete Edwards regards as common sense. And his credentials speak volumes. A fully qualified fitness instructor (or 'preparator' as he prefers to be known), he studied Italian training methods at first hand for a number of years.

He was so impressed, and intrigued, by the Italian training methods that he is now introducing those same ideals into the British game. Having worked with the professionals at Arsenal, Luton and Leyton Orient, he has been a key member of the Nottingham Forest coaching staff. It is his responsibility to ensure every player he works with is physically prepared to his peak to endure the rigours of a typical English football season.

From the first, painful stretches of the pre-season build-up to the last kick of the final game he works out training routines for both the team and the players as individuals. He also arranges their everyday diet; another increasingly important aspect of a footballer's preparation.

His aims are simple – to make sure footballers can perform at their peak for the full 90 minutes of a match. If they are not properly prepared, players don't enjoy the game and supporters will not be entertained. He says:

'It is my belief that the best Italian methods can be used throughout the world to develop players at all levels and enable them to make the most of their talent. In my work at pro level, I have taken the methods of some of the very best Italian preparators and adapted them to complement the physical and technical abilities of British players.

'I worked with the first team squad at Arsenal when they were regarded as one of the fittest and most complete sides in the game. It was with that in mind that I went to Italy to study training and preparation methods. The difference in standards and fitness was staggering. I built a rapport with several top trainers and have kept in touch with these people ever since to keep up with the latest practices. I've introduced these methods to great effect at Premier League level, and they now form the basis of this book.

'It has taken time to break down barriers, but positive steps have now been taken and this book takes the process one step further. The thing that struck me most as I continued to compare the performances of players in Italy and England, was the superior fitness of the Italians over a period of 90 minutes. The pressure they apply on and off the ball throughout a game is very impressive. I didn't feel British players at that time could do it to the same degree. But I felt if the British could develop that side of their game, they could be up there with the best teams in the world.

'I have already taken steps in the right direction but what we have achieved is merely the tip of the iceberg. We have seen the benefits of players training and preparing for games to their maximum capacity. Others could, and should, follow suit. Not least in their pre-season routines which, invariably, involve lots of running and very little work without the ball. So many players pick up injuries at this time because of over-intensive training methods and these should be avoided. There are so many things managers and coaches – and of course the players themselves – can do to get more out of individuals. Hopefully this book will go some way towards helping you achieve your own peak football fitness.

Good luck!'

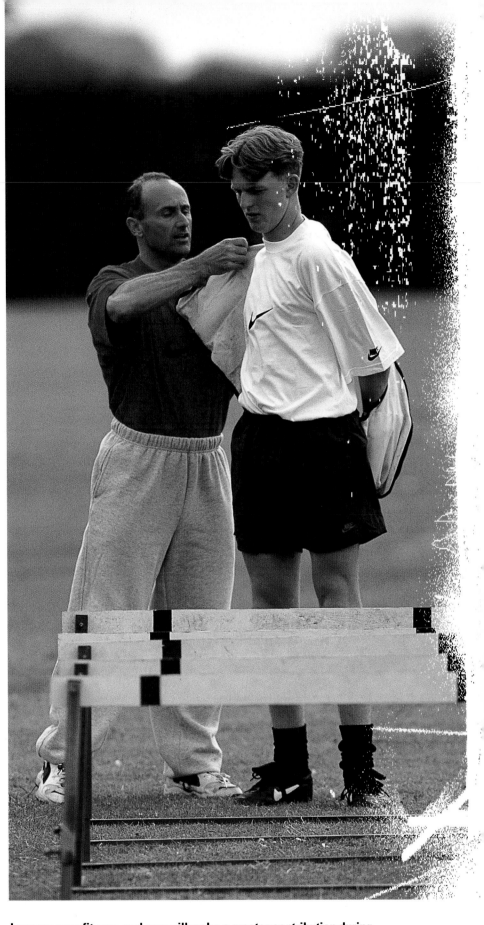

Improve your fitness, and you will make a greater contribution during matches. But take care to work on all areas of fitness.
Here, a young player prepares for a high-intensity session, which will improve his explosive fitness.

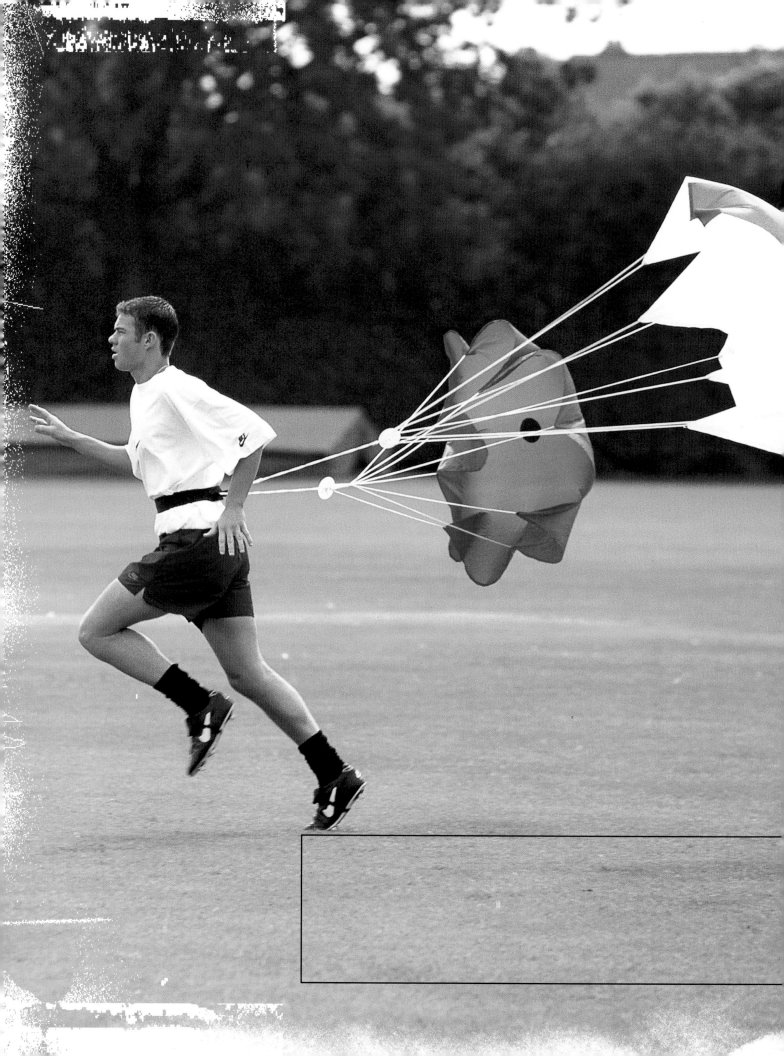

1

fitness

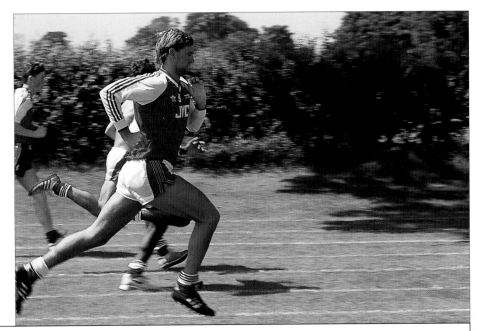

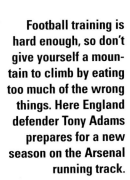

Football training is hard enough, so don't give yourself a mountain to climb by eating too much of the wrong things. Here England defender Tony Adams prepares for a new season on the Arsenal running track.

If you don't eat the right things — at the right time — you cannot get the best out of your body. Simple advice, but a message worth remembering if you're serious about preparing yourself for the exertions of training and playing. To achieve the best possible results it is important to follow a strict dietary code. Sure, let yourself go every now and again by tucking into a rich, slap-up meal. But don't do anything to excess and enjoy your 'treats' in moderation. For a number of years, players in Italy have enjoyed specially designed diets according to their individual needs. This is something which has been introduced throughout Europe in recent years. Remarkable progress has been made in educating players as to the importance of diet and, nowadays, players are much more sensible about what they eat — both while at their club and at home.

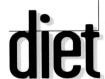

diet

STRIKING A BALANCE

The days of steak and eggs for a pre-match meal and fish and chips as a post-match top-up are long gone. Most football clubs now insist on their players eating pasta, rice, chicken or fish as part of their big game preparation. The important thing to consider – and the key to achieving peak fitness – is striking the right balance between your in-take of carbohydrates, fat and protein.

Fat has double the calories of carbohydrate and protein but that doesn't mean it gives you more energy. Nothing, in fact, could be further from the truth. Fat in itself is something the body uses slowly – storing any surplus in various parts of the body. Protein also takes a long time for the body to utilise but, just like fat, it is an essential component of a healthy diet. The most important things a footballer can eat are carbohydrates. And we will be explaining more about them in the next few pages.

FILLING YOUR TANKS

Training and playing are basically the same when it comes to fuelling the body. Eat the wrong food and you can't train hard enough to prepare yourself for playing. The two things go hand in hand. Without the right fuel you are not going to play to your full potential. It's like putting low-grade fuel in a high performance car – the two don't mix and the results are disappointing. The importance of having a good diet cannot be emphasised highly enough, so take a good look at your eating habits and find the areas for improvement. You will be surprised by the results.

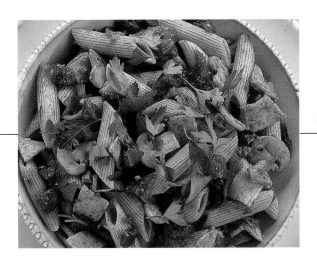

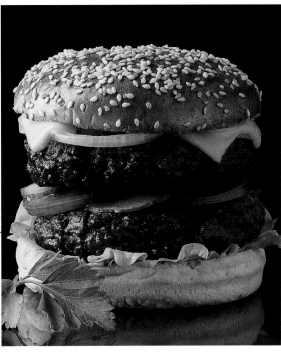

Far left: Pasta has become the staple food of the modern athlete. It is an excellent source of carbohydrate...not to mention a versatile and tasty food.

Left: All things in moderation, even burgers. But don't let treats dominate your diet. The more fatty foods you eat, the more you'll have to train.

CARBOHYDRATES AND PROTEINS

As we explained briefly above, carbohydrates are the most important part of an athlete's diet. Without them he or she can't function; it's as simple as that. There are two types of carbohydrate: simple and complex. Simple carbs are derived from dried fruits and sugars. They should only complement, not replace, the more important, complex carbs which provide a quicker source of energy and are found in starchy foods like potatoes and whole grain products, including flour, bread and pasta.

A common myth is that proteins give you energy. But this is a fallacy. Proteins take too long to digest to be a valuable source of quick energy. The role of proteins is, in fact, to build and maintain muscle. For this reason, they are an important part of your overall diet. You cannot, and should not, avoid eating all fat, but as an athlete fats must not dominate your diet.

The right food stuffs, eaten at the right time, will provide you with the extra glycogen which can make all the difference. Diet can improve your performances but you have to eat the right things consistently to get real benefits.

know your food groups

Everyone knows they should eat a healthy balanced diet. But what exactly is a 'healthy balanced diet.'

If you know you don't eat a balanced diet, make the effort and keep yourself healthy by taking regular supplements. There are many different types available, including special varieties for athletes and vegetarians.

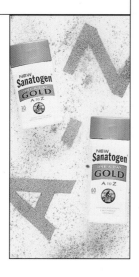

CARBOHYDRATES

Carbohydrate is the fuel on which your body runs. It is stored in your liver and muscles as a substance called glycogen. Good sources of carbohydrate include potatoes, pasta, rice and bread. These are converted to glycogen which is stored in the liver and to a lesser extent the muscles until it is carried in the blood to muscle cells during exercise. There it is burned up to produce energy. Carbohydrate is easy to digest and has a high water content, making it particularly useful when eaten before or even during exercise. The relative calories (and therefore food) burned during activity depend on the fitness and metabolism of the individual and the intensity and duration of the exercise. To be sure you have plenty of carbohydrate available for your glycogen stores, you should eat regular meals. Particularly in the three days leading up to a match, players should eat four small meals a day. Don't skip a meal and then binge later.

PROTEINS

Protein is used for building muscle and is vital for growth and to maintain health. But, because it takes a long time to digest, it is not a source of immediate energy. You need a regular supply of protein, although not as much as you might think. You don't want protein with lots of fat (such as red meat and dairy products). Better protein sources are white poultry meat, fish and soya beans. Protein requirements do not rise significantly with heavy exercise, so your intake should remain constant. Meat is synonymous with protein, but there are many other sources – particularly fish and soya – which are higher in protein and are lower in fat than meat.

SUPPLEMENTS

Providing you eat plenty of fresh fruit and vegetables, you do not need to worry about vitamins. The vitamins you need plenty of are A (found in vegetables including spinach, carrots, sweet corn), C (found in fruit and fruit juice) and E (found in nuts, seeds and whole grains).

If you feel the need to supplement your diet you can do so with extra vitamins in the form of tablets or 'local' carbs or proteins in the form of powder mixed with liquid.

The time to do this would be if you miss a meal, but don't make a habit of it – the best way to obtain these vitamins is through fruit and vegetables. Tablets are there as a supplement not a substitute. Apart from vitamin supplements, some of the products on the market have been shown to produce good results, particularly in strength. Remember, these are not drugs but supplements available from chemists. However, all youngsters should check with their parents before taking tablets of any kind.

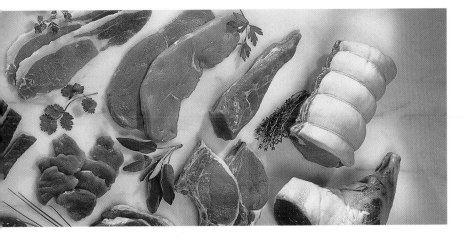

◀ PROTEIN SOURCES

- Meat
- Fish
- Cheese
- Eggs
- Soya
- Nuts

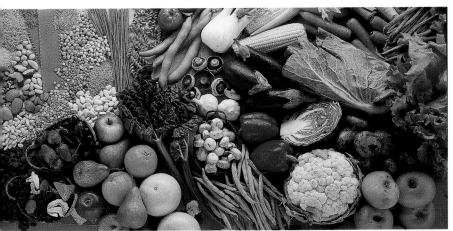

◀ CARBOHYDRATE SOURCES

- Potatoes
- Cereals and other whole grain products
- Rice
- Pasta
- Food made with flour
- Food made with sugar
- Dried fruit
- Vegetables

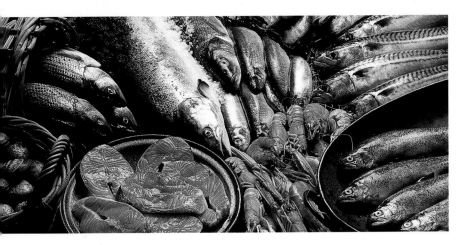

◀ FAT SOURCES

- Milk products
- Nuts
- Fish
- Meat

DO...

...increase your complex carbohydrates – bread, potatoes, rice, pasta etc.– three days before playing

...drink isotonic drinks free from sodium

...eat within four hours of playing or training

...eat the right foods before training...not just when you're playing a match

DON'T...

...take in excess fat or salt or drink alcohol prior to a game

...eat burgers, chocolate or anything containing saturated fat

...add fat to your food e.g. butter on jacket potatoes

...drink tea or coffee at half-time – they are both diuretic and drain fluid rather than replace it

eat to play

If you eat the wrong things three days before a game it can be just as harmful to your performance as a poor pre-match meal. On the other hand, if you eat plenty of carbohydrates three days before a game your muscles will be fuelled when you come to play. However, you must eat the right kind of carbohydrates. Complex carbohydrates with little in the way of fat or protein should be eaten for the three days prior to the game. On the day of the game itself, you should concentrate on eating carbs that will give you instant fuel. Even canned fruit can give you valuable energy. Popular foods include light pasta — but avoid rich sauces — cereal and whole grain products and dried fruits.

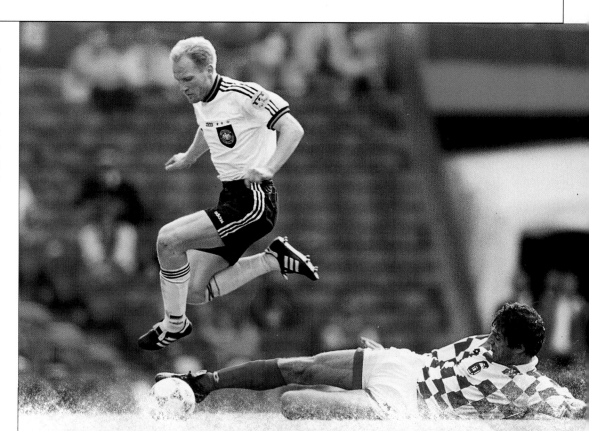

To compete at the very top level, players like Matthias Sammer and Slaven Bilic have to make sure that they have eaten the right types of food. If they don't, they will not have the fuel in their tanks to keep going for 90 minutes.

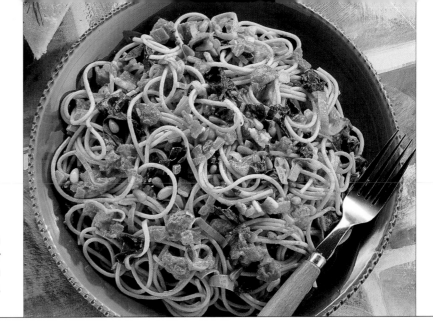

Carbohydrates should dominate an athlete's diet. Pasta is a popular choice, but avoid sauces which contain a lot of sugar.

A PROFESSIONAL DIET

A good pre-match meal counts for nothing if your diet is poor for the rest of the week. Professional footballers have to be disciplined with their food, but they don't have to live like monks. You can go out and have a decent meal in the evening providing the rest of your day you haven't been eating rubbish. It is all about educating people to eat well and know what's good and what's bad for them. A healthy diet for a professional footballer should contain plenty of carbohydrate, for example:

Breakfast
Cereal, half a pint of skimmed milk, bread and preserve. Tea or coffee and orange juice.

Lunch (after training)
A meal high in complex carbohydrates with a small intake of protein. Chicken with rice or jacket potato and green vegetables. Pasta is also popular. This will be followed by fruit and an isotonic drink. On the occasions that British footballers train in the afternoon their lunch is a lighter meal with simple carbs like pasta and fruit. Again isotonic drink to boost.

Evening Meal
A meal high in complex carbohydrates with a small intake of protein. Chicken with rice or jacket potato and green vegetables. Pasta is also popular. This will be followed by fruit and an isotonic drink. On the occasions that British footballers train in the afternoon their lunch is a lighter meal with simple carbs like pasta and fruit. Again isotonic drink to boost.

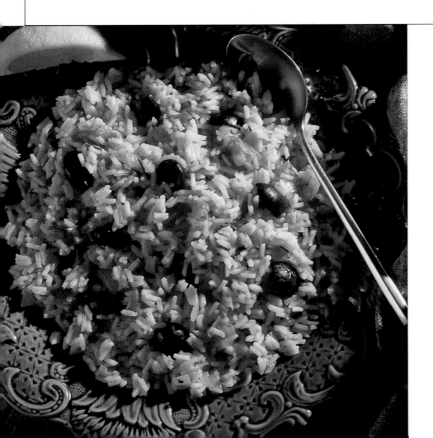

◄ CARBO LOADING

• Three days prior to playing start carbo loading which means that 75% of what you eat during that period should be complex carbohydrates from the range listed, including the dried fruits and cereals. Try to eat four small meals a day rather than two big meals. Your body absorbs smaller amounts much easier than huge portions

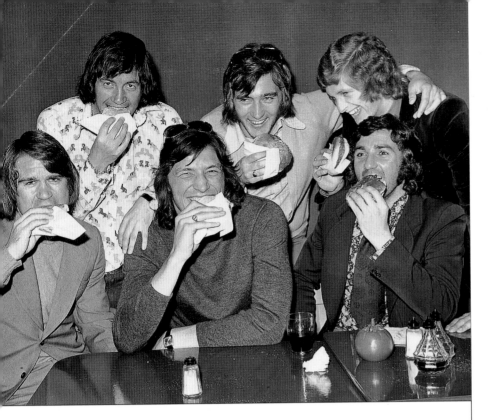

Until recently, footballers at all levels of the game were happy to eat what they liked when they liked. The picture (left) shows Chelsea players tucking into hamburgers in 1972. Nowadays top professionals are more likely to be sampling Italian cuisine than such fatty fare.

A player who eats the right things (plenty of carbohydrates) at the right times (regular, small meals) has plenty of energy to play football. By contrast, a player who fasts during the day and binges on a slap-up meal at night takes on calories at the wrong time and has little energy to play football the next day. Different players react in different ways to particular foods and mealtimes. All athletes must get to know their own body and its needs. However, you must maintain a balanced diet and not eat any one thing to excess. It is about striking a balance; doing things in moderation.

keep your tanks full

REPLENISHMENT

A high carbohydrate diet provides players with greater glycogen stores and the energy to keep going at the end of a game. No matter how aerobically fit you are, if there is no fuel in the tank you will run out of energy. The only way to keep your tanks topped up is to eat, but you must eat the right things at the right times. Diet is critical.

But, even if you have prepared well and eaten the right things prior to the game, you will still need to watch your diet after exercise. Research has shown that footballers' glycogen levels can be down as much as 75% after a game and those levels have to be restored to normal as soon as possible.

Post-match meals have, traditionally, consisted of a few drinks in the bar and fish and chips on the coach. There are stacks of calories in this sort of food, but it is not the best way to get your glycogen store back up.

It is just as important to eat the right things after a game as it is in the build-up. At top professional clubs, a chef travels everywhere with the team. He, or she, ensures that players eat the correct foods both before and after a match. You have two to five hours to replace your glycogen stores after a game and it is crucial that you eat the right things. Try to eat plenty of carbohydrates after the game (pasta is particularly good); eating junk food will undo all of your good pre-match preparation.

Ideally, players should eat within two hours of a game finishing. Some players don't want to eat after exercise, but you must condition your body and make post-match refuelling part of your routine.

Beer is often consumed as a traditional post-match celebration. However, drinking alcohol after a match is ill-advised. Firstly, alcohol is a diuretic and so dehydrates you at a time when your body is in need of rehydration. And secondly, alcohol suppresses your appetite, thus preventing you from replacing much needed glycogen stores. It all hinders your recovery from the exertions of the match.

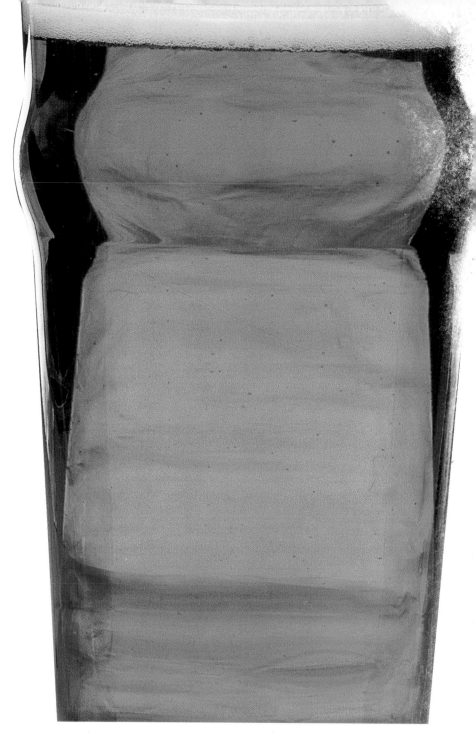

PIGGING OUT

It is okay to deviate from the perfect athletes' diet every now and then. But, overall you should be eating the right things at the right time. If you eat fish and chips you must balance it with a strict diet over the next couple of days. All things in moderation. The thing to remember is that everything you eat has a consequence – some good, some bad. Eat the wrong things at the wrong times and you will have to pay the price, either with your diet over the subsequent days, or on the pitch.

FLUIDS

The human body is made up of 80% fluid. Every time you exercise fluid is lost and, to keep healthy and fit, these fluids must be replaced. Footballers should drink at least half a litre of water before and after a warm-up. It is also a good idea to consume an isotonic drink before playing a game.

ISOTONIC DRINKS

Isotonic drinks are easily absorbed into the blood stream and provide quicker rehydration than water. There are many specially designed isotonic drinks on the market, but a simple isotonic solution can be made by mixing equal quantities of fruit juice and water. Try to drink before you become thirsty. Once you have reached this point, you will have already become sluggish and your blood will have thickened.

ALCOHOLIC DRINKS

Just as eating the wrong things after exercise affects your performance, so too does drinking the wrong sorts of fluids. The consumption of alcohol following a game is particularly damaging to a footballer's fitness. Players traditionally head straight to the bar after a game, but this is the worst thing they can do. After a game players are naturally dehydrated and need to take on fluids quickly, but alcohol is a diuretic and dehydrates players still further. Drinking alcohol suppresses your hunger so you can go longer without eating anything to replace the glycogen stores. All the time you are drinking alcohol, you are putting your recovery period back.

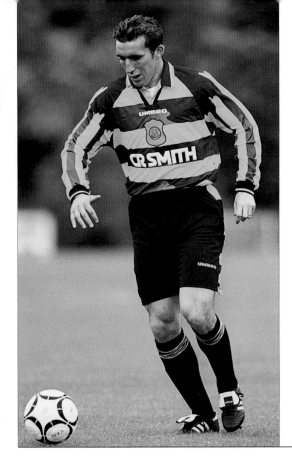

Hard pitches and hot weather can make pre-season friendlies gruelling. They are, however, essential if you want to achieve a good level of match fitness. Here Alan Stubbs of Celtic prepares for the start of the season at a non-League ground.

achieving base fitness

Ask any player to name the worst thing about being a professional footballer and the answer, virtually to a man, is...pre-season training. You've just had six weeks off, perhaps spent on a sun-drenched isle, and all of a sudden a sergeant-major figure is putting you through your paces. Your head's pounding, lungs bursting and legs screaming for help. It's the time of year every player hates.

But things could be a lot easier for many players – if they looked after their bodies a little better during the summer recess. Coaches and managers hope that when a player begins pre-season training he will be in a reasonable condition. Professional players are all given a programme – relating to both diet and fitness – to follow which should enable them to report back with their bodies in good, physical order. A typical programme will allow players a reasonable break from all exercise and should be started around three weeks prior to pre-season proper begins.

If players follow their programmes, the coaching staff will be working with players who have a decent base level of fitness...and not working from scratch.

Footballers at all levels should keep themselves ticking over during the summer. If you keep relatively fit, the new season will not seem so daunting. If you don't have a decent level of base fitness, you will not achieve full match fitness. You will strive too hard to reach the next level and pick up injuries as a result. You can end up going backwards.

LEVEL 1

Assuming players maintain a decent level of fitness, pre-season training will concentrate on raising fitness levels through relatively easy, daily runs combined with stretching and strengthening exercises. These exercises will strengthen the tendons, ligaments and joints before the hard work really begins.

LEVEL 2

In the professional game, Level 1 training will continue for around seven days. Training will then move players on to the next level of base fitness. Emphasis is placed on bringing the oxygen levels up and making greater demands of the body. Similar exercises are used to those in Level 1, but everything is done at a slightly quicker rate. That's how a player's base level of fitness is determined. Once that has been achieved the real work can begin.

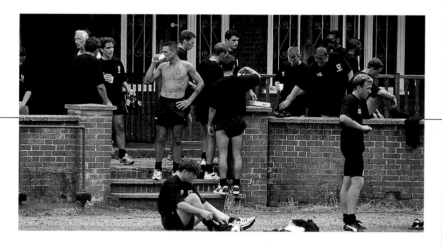

PRE-SEASON AIMS

During a competitive football match, a player works at a rate in excess of 75% of his maximum fitness level. Pre-season training needs to progress to reflect this level of work – even exaggerating it at certain points. Four weeks into pre-season training, the trainer should be looking to work players as if they are playing in a game.

RECOVERY DURING PRE-SEASON

It is important to allow your body adequate time to recover between sessions during pre-season. You can't do a long run one day and then expect to go out and do an even longer run the next. It doesn't work that way. You have to do things over an eight-day period with sufficient rest between. A common problem is that players try to top up their fitness programme daily. All they do is come to a point where they are so fatigued that they go backwards. Give yourself adequate time to recover.

PART-TIME PRE-SEASON

Part-time players should raise their fitness by training, initially, for three nights a week. Work rate should be increased from a 20-minute run on the first day's training to a 30-minute run three nights later. You would increase the duration of the exercise as a professional would, but it obviously takes longer to reach a similar level of fitness. The same principles of allowing the body time to recover from each session still apply.

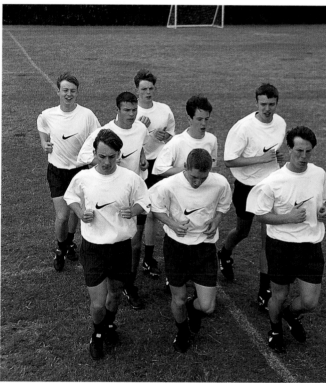

Running (above) is an essential part of pre-season training. To achieve a high level of fitness, exercise must be combined with appropriate recovery periods, as demonstrated by Wimbledon FC (left).

SUMMER TIP

• Low-impact aerobic exercise can break the monotony of training during the summer. Cycling and swimming are excellent ways to keep fit and involve very low risk of injury. Keep a close eye on your weight and three weeks before returning to football step up your own personal training programme

Short, high-intensity runs are an important part of pre-season training. Each run should be followed by a period of recovery. Here, players sprint for 25 yards, turn and walk back for 25 yards (recovery) and then repeat six times. (See also the exercise opposite.)

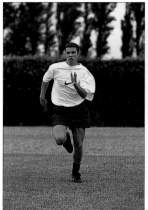
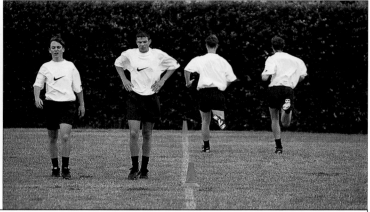

Once you have achieved a base level of fitness, the priority should be to build lung and aerobic capacity and develop the strength and power in the leg muscles. This is when the dreaded hill work starts.

improving pre-season fitness

DISTANCE RUNNING

You do not need to be able to run a marathon to be fit for football. In most cases, it is better to run a shorter distance at a greater pace than to set off on a time-consuming long jog. Try to run at a pace that increases your fitness level. For stamina work, players should start off running 3,000m and work up to 8,000m. Repeats of 300, 600 and 900m runs are also useful. A professional session might involve running three repeats of 900m, followed by three repeats of 600m and finished off with three repeats of 300m. Each run would be separated by a 2.5-minute break.

This type of running should be punctuated with ball work – ideally small-sided games. The running and the practice game should complement one another – if the running is high intensity (see page 56) then the game should be moderate intensity (see p60) and vice versa. Whichever combination you choose, make sure the lower intensity work is done last as this can form part of the overall warm-down.

HILL RUNNING

Find a hill which really works your leg muscles when you run up it, but don't go for a monster – a 30% gradient will only demoralise you. When you've settled on a hill, run short repeats. Hill repeats of between eight and 21 seconds are recommended. The following schedule will provide a vigorous work-out (a schedule based on half the number of repeats would be ideal for most amateur players):

- 6 x 21-second repeats
- 6 x 15-second repeats
- 6 x 12-second repeats
- 6 x 10-second repeats
- 6 x 8-second repeats

When you have achieved a decent base level of fitness, you can safely increase your speed, as you progress through the repeats, without risking injury. It is essential to stretch properly before hill work. It is an exercise that puts a great strain on your body, so prepare properly.

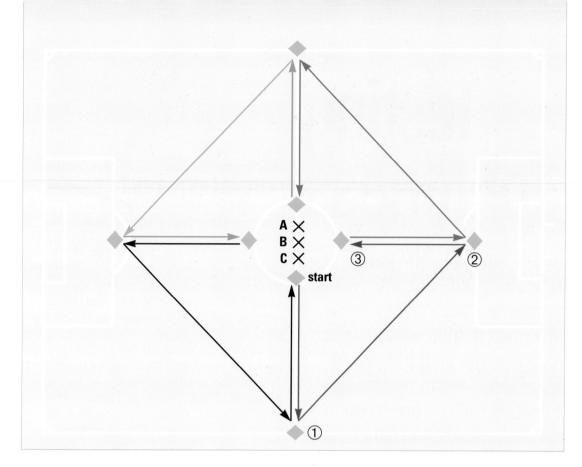

Player A sets off sprinting for mark ① when he gets there player **B** sets off, when **B** reaches mark ① player **C** sets off. All players continue their runs unbroken to mark ③.
As soon as all three players are at mark ③ they set off on run two. This exercise is repeated until all players are back at start.

SPEED TRAINING

Once players have attained a good level of stamina, the aim should be to improve their speed. This is done through a combination of high-intensity small-sided games and high-intensity running. The aim is to improve the leg power, the strength of the muscles and aerobic capacity. For more information on this sort of training, see page 56. Specially designed parachutes and weighted jackets are particularly useful for this type of training.

ASSESSING FITNESS

As soon as players seem to have attained a good level of speed and stamina they can be assessed in games over a 90-minute period. If they cannot get through the full length of a match then return to the stamina training. If, however, players have achieved the sort of fitness levels required to get them through 90 minutes to an acceptable standard, the work can be stepped up still further, introducing shorter, sharper running. This type of work can be done both with and without the ball.

PREPARING FOR POSITIONS

It is also at this stage that players should be separated out according to their positions. Their fitness must be honed according to their role within the team. Midfielders do more running during a game than defenders or strikers so their level of fitness and stamina has to be slightly higher. Defenders need a great deal of strength and strikers need to develop their acceleration and overall pace.

PRE-SEASON FRIENDLIES

No team should go into a new season without any match practice, but pre-season friendlies are important not only for getting tactics right, but also for gauging fitness. It may even be the case that a player's fitness, in relation to his team-mates, dictates his role within the team. Playing games will obviously help to improve fitness levels, but basic fitness cannot be achieved without training, in the main, without the ball.

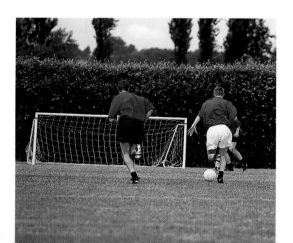

Playing practice matches in training is an excellent way to improve your fitness. It also gives you the opportunity to develop tactics for the season to come.

testing for fitness

A runner can gauge his fitness by the times he records in his particular event, but with footballers, it's not that straightforward. Players themselves are the best judges of their own fitness, although invariably it's left to the coach to recognise the fitness levels of those under his charge. In most cases his decision will be based upon nothing more than performances in matches. In clear-cut cases, for instance where a player flags in the last 15 minutes of a game in which he hasn't worked particularly hard, it is easy for the coach to conclude that his fitness level is not up to scratch. In such a case, training programmes should be revised to get fitness levels back up to an appropriate level as quickly as possible. However, it is far better to assess fitness before players get into match situations. The coach will undoubtedly form opinions about what he sees during a match or training, but a variety of tests can be used to back up his judgement.

THE BLEEP TEST

The most common fitness test used by football clubs is the bleep test. Two cones are set 20 metres apart and an audio bleep recorder is set at one end. This device makes a bleep sound a set number of times per minute. The sound is used to pace the player being tested. The pace of the bleep gets progressively faster and as it speeds up, the player has to make more and more runs per minute. The player continues until he can complete no more 20-metre runs within the time between bleeps. His result is determined by the level (i.e. the number of bleeps per minute) at which he had to stop. Results are between one and 21. A player with a good level of fitness should achieve a score of around level 15 or 16.

BENEFITS OF THE BLEEP

The bleep test provides an insight into how far advanced a player is in his own particular training programme. It can't tell everything about a player's level of fitness but it is a useful guide. Most importantly it helps a player understand more about his own fitness and realise when he has reached a certain level.

This self-analysis can be a good motivating factor. For example, if a player records a bleep test score of 16 and then subsequently registers 17 or 18, he will feel good about his fitness. By the same token, if he records a 16 followed by a 14 he will recognise the need to work himself harder in order to halt and then rectify his falling standards.

The test also introduces a competitive element to a club's training programme. The fittest players often battle it out for the highest score and top slot, while players at the other end of the scale will not wish to be regarded as the worst trainers at the club.

WHEN TO USE THE BLEEP TEST

The bleep test is employed to assess fitness at a number of points during the season. It is first used during early pre-season training in order to gauge players' physical state after the summer break. Players should be retested just before the start of the playing season and their progress assessed. A suitable programme of training should then be devised.

The test is also useful when assessing the recovery rate of a player who is rehabilitating from an injury.

A run of poor results may also lead to a session of testing. Poor fitness is often the cause of poor form. If you can determine where the problem lies you can take action to remedy it. A new schedule will need to be drawn up as a result of the test results. Two or three weeks into this new schedule, the test should be repeated to see if things are improving

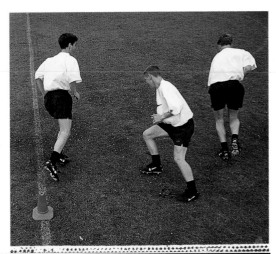

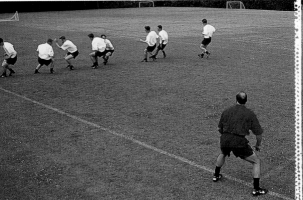

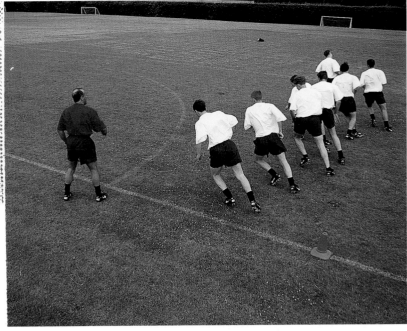

The bleep test helps coaches assess the fitness of players and develop training sessions to improve fitness where necessary. The players start running between cones and are paced by a bleep sound. The bleeps get progressively faster and the players must speed up accordingly until each of them is forced to stop.

A pulse monitor is an excellent aid for fitness training. Basic models aren't too expensive. The only function you need is the pulse display, though some models have alarms that sound if your pulse goes above or below a particular level.

PULSE MONITOR

The most useful aid to individual training is a pulse monitor. These devices have been used for many years in both cycling and athletics. Basic models are relatively inexpensive and simply provide a pulse display from which you can take constant readings. Some models have alarms which bleep if your pulse drops below, or rises above, certain levels. Alternatively, you can take your own pulse by placing two fingers on your wrist and counting the number of beats in a minute. Try this after exercise to gauge your rate of recovery.

Goalkeepers must be extremely supple. They have to be ready, at all times, to throw themselves at shots and crosses to protect their goal. Here, Erik Thorstvedt arches his back and diverts a goal-bound shot.

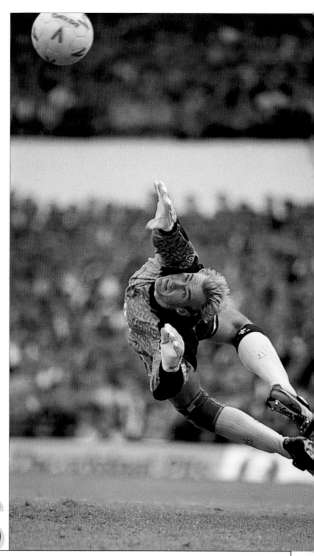

suppleness

Whether you're warming-up before a game or before a basic training session, take great care to stretch properly and ensure your body is supple enough to perform at its peak. It is also essential to warm-down after exercise. If you don't warm-up and stretch properly before a game — especially on a cold day — you run a high risk of injury and the possibility of being sidelined for weeks or even months. All for the sake of a few minutes preparing your body for the hard work that is to follow. Is it worth the risk? Of course it's not. Remember, if you injure yourself, you'll lose your fitness and have to go through all the stamina and strength training outlined in the pre-season section.

Frenchman Christian Karembeu stretches every sinew in his right leg to dispossess Romanian Dorinel Munteanu. A tackle like this puts tremendous strain on muscles and ligaments and, without proper warming-up, can result in injury.

LEARN FROM THE PROS

Throughout the professional game, and in particular in Europe, warming-up is taken very seriously. Prepare properly and you give yourself a better chance of performing to the best of your ability for the duration of a game. Whatever level you play at, there is no reason why you can't go through a short but thorough warm-up and stretching routine.

STRETCH TO PLAY

Warming-up for a training session or match should start with light stretching (see exercises on following pages) for 15 minutes. This should be followed by light running which will get the body temperature and the heart rate up. This primes the muscles for a quick start. Continue the warm-up until you are breathing quite heavily and the muscles are fully stretched. At this point, you will be ready to go into a game, or begin a high or moderate intensity training session, with the risk of unnecessary injury diminished.

PRE-SEASON WARM-UPS

A great deal of emphasis is placed on warming-up nowadays. Even so, pre-season injuries, due to poor warming-up are still all too common (even at the very top level of the game). Injuries at this stage, for whatever reason, are costly as players will fail to reach their maximum fitness level for the start of the season. It is easy to be overkeen during pre-season, but it is essential to take your time and prepare properly for the season's early exertions. If you rush your preparation, the results can be disastrous.

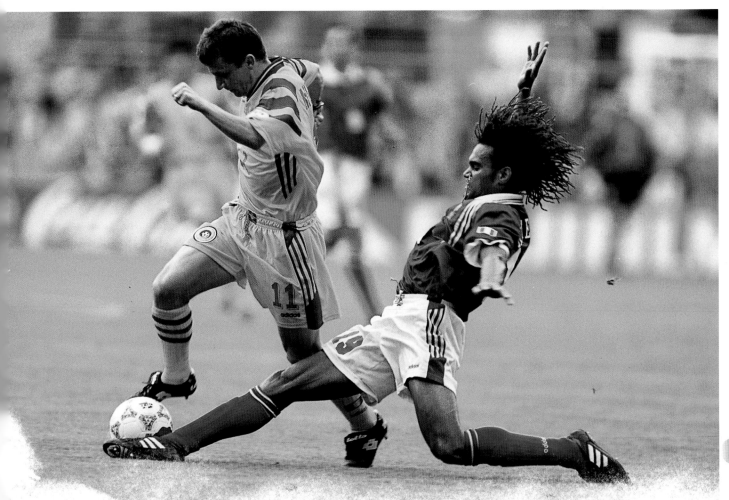

upper body and hips

Legs are an outfield player's most important tools. But when warming up don't forget the top half of your body. It is vital that the whole body is warm, supple and prepared for exercise. A 'top to bottom' warm-up — starting with the upper body and hips, and finishing with the calf and Achilles — is the best way to get your body properly prepared for the rigours of exercise.
Before you begin any stretching, however, it is advisable to jog gently around the pitch or training field for a few minutes to raise the body temperature and your heart rate. Don't do anything excessive and always remember you shouldn't stretch a muscle which is cold.

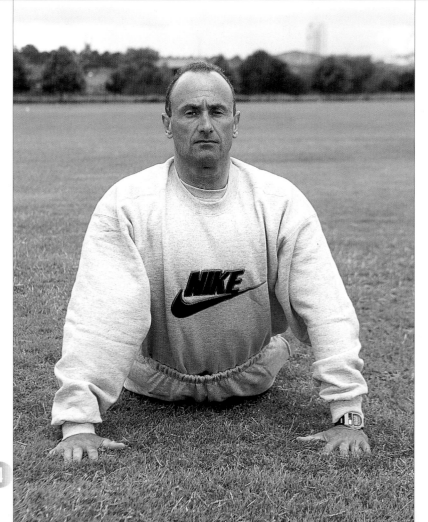

◄ STRETCH TO PLAY

This exercise stretches the abdomen (the stomach and hips). It also benefits the lower back and give the triceps in the back of the arm a good stretch too. The arms should be spread slightly more than shoulder width apart. Push up gently into the position shown and hold for a few seconds. Repeat ten times.

▶ SIDE BEND

There are many variations of the side bend exercise and this is one of the most effective. It stretches the side, the tricep muscle and the upper lats (latissimus dorsi muscle). It also helps to stretch the abdomen and, by using the arm as demonstrated, the frontal deltoid muscle. It is a truly multi-functional exercise.

Stand with your legs 2ft (approximately 60cm) apart, place one arm above your head and the other behind your back and bend to the side as shown. Don't bend forward or back. Your movement should be slow and gentle. When you feel the tension, hold the stretch for between 15 and 20 seconds. Repeat the exercise on the other side.

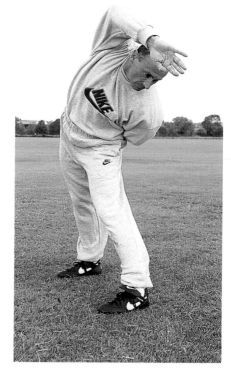
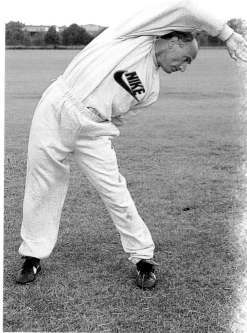

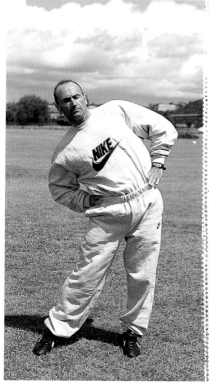
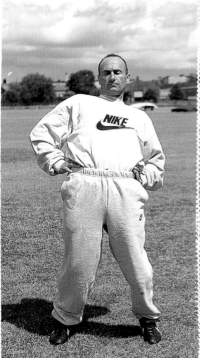
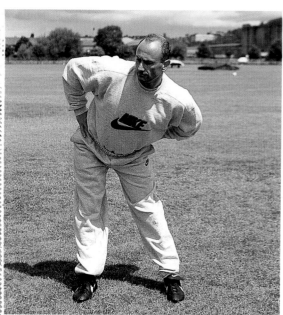

▲ HIP ROLL

The hips give your body a wide range of movement. Injuries of the hip joint are rare in sport (although wear and tear arthritis can occur in older sportsmen) but it is important to warm this area properly before serious exercise.

Try to achieve a rolling motion, pushing the hip out to the left, out to the front and all the way round to complete a full circle. Do this five or six times, rotating your hips one way and then switching to roll them the other.

TIPS

- Avoid sharp, sudden movements. Keep your stretching smooth and you won't get injured in the warm-up
- Always perform exercises slowly and do not over-stretch yourself. Hold the position and then repeat
- Breathe through your nose and continue to exhale and inhale as you work through the exercise. Do not hold your breath at any point druing the exercise
- Stop immediately if you feel any sharp pain

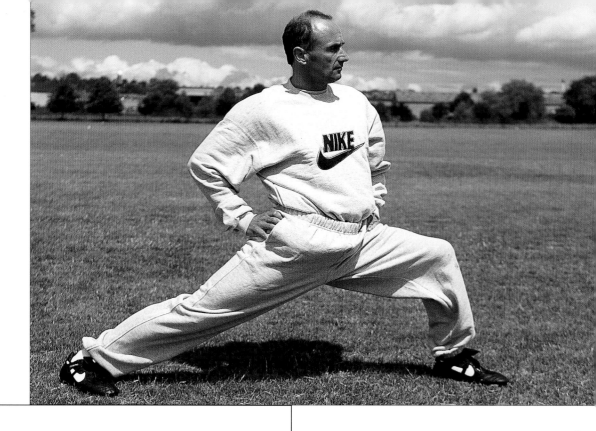

Soccer players, more than most sportsmen, are susceptible to groin strains. The groin muscles, which are located on the inside of the thigh, can be damaged when a player over-stretches, or stretches awkwardly, for a ball or tackle. In some cases groin injuries are unavoidable. But the better you prepare your body the greater the chances of avoiding injury — and the better your chances of a quick recovery should it happen. It is also worth noting that most muscle injuries occur during the first 15 minutes of each half. So remember is it important not only to warm-up thoroughly before a game, but also to keep your muscles warm during half-time, particularly the groin and hamstrings.

lower body

▲ THE GROIN AND MORE

This exercise works several muscles. The inner groin, calves and ankles all receive benefits from this basic stretch. Adopt the position shown in the picture, with your leading leg at an angle of almost 90 degrees to the ground and the other leg stretched behind. Put your hands on hips and hold a stable position for ten seconds and then change.

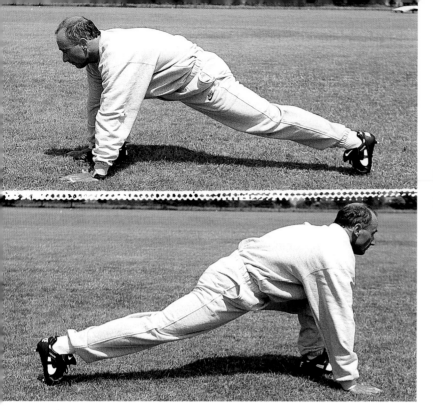

◀ ON YOUR MARKS

This is an exaggerated version of a sprinter's starting position. The following muscles are stretched by this exercise – frontal groin area, thigh, calf and Achilles. Adopt the position of an elevated press-up, with your arms shoulder width apart for support, and then bring one foot up between your hands. Dip your body weight towards the ground from the waist. Hold and repeat bringing your other foot forward. This is a good exercise to start with before moving on to the advanced stretches illustrated below.

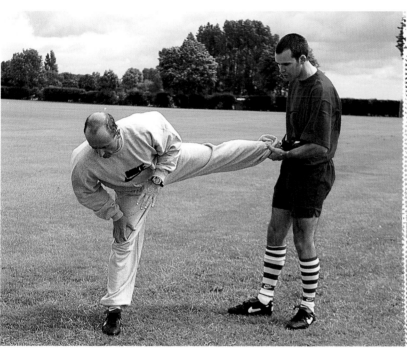

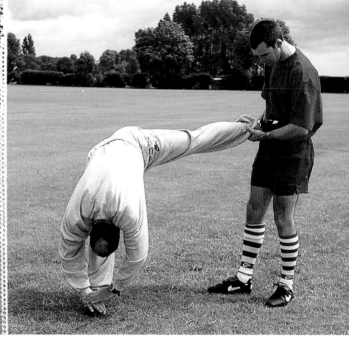

TIPS

- The advanced stretch should only be attempted when you have carried out the other groin exercises
- Always hold a stable, balanced body position. Uneven weight distribution will make exercises more difficult and, often, less effective
- Do not position your arms or legs too far apart, otherwise you may lose your balance
- Don't rush into any of the stretches. Ease yourself into them gently and listen to your body

▲ ADVANCED STRETCH

You need good flexibility and a partner to attempt this exercise. It should only ever be carried out when you have completed the groin stretch above. It works the inner groin and the inner section of the quad muscle of the leg being held and the hamstring of the standing leg. Once you are comfortable with your starting position (left), slowly bend forward and try to touch your toes.

hamstring

The hamstring (or the rear leg biceps to be more accurate) is located at the back of the leg. It is a muscle group which travels all the way from the lower buttock to the back of the knee.
As anyone who has suffered a hamstring tear (sprint athletes and speedy wingers are particularly susceptible) will tell you, this injury is extremely painful.
Imagine the pain of a red hot needle being stuck into the back of your leg. Hamstring injuries always occur suddenly (it's like an elastic band snapping) and, while there can be no guaranteed protection, good stretching is the soundest precaution you can take. It will also make you more flexible, helping you get into more exaggerated positions.
Most hamstring injuries occur when the muscles are not sufficiently warm to cope with a sudden, explosive burst of speed — often in the opening stages of matches.

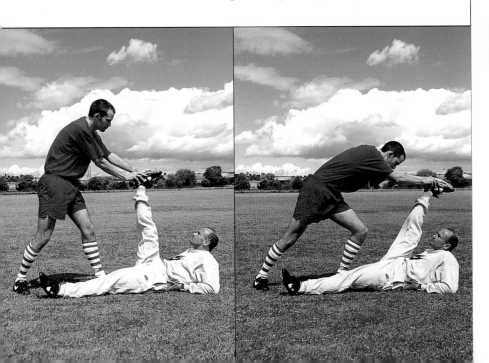

◄ ASSISTED STRETCH

Another assisted and advanced stretch, using your elbows for support. Raise the working leg to 90 degrees and hold. With the aid of your partner, gradually bring your leg (keeping it straight at all times) towards you. Hold for six seconds and repeat, pushing the leg that bit further each time until you are at full stretch. Keep the resting leg flat to the floor. Remember, this is an advanced exercise for flexible people.

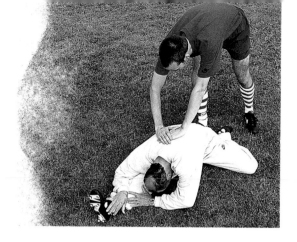

◄ THE HURDLE STRETCH

This can be done in the early stages of a warm-up. Tuck the non-working leg under your backside and stretch the other leg out in front of you as shown. Put your head down towards your knee and reach out with both hands towards the ankle. Feel the tension and hold. Repeat. For an advanced version of this exercise, get a partner to apply downward pressure on your back. This will take your head lower and your hands further.

► DEEP HAMSTRING STRETCH

This exercise stretches the leg which is held by your partner. Start with your legs at 90 degrees to each other, your body upright and hands on hips for extra balance. Gradually push your head down towards your knee, with your hands around the ankle as shown for a deep, hamstring stretch.

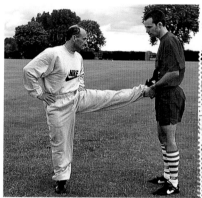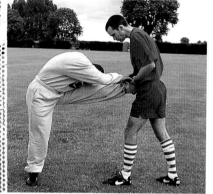

▼ THE FLOOR SPLIT

This is an advanced exercise which many people will be unable to complete fully. If that is the case, start with your legs closer together and only take your head down a short way. Gradually widen your legs, pushing your head down towards the ground (top) or towards your knees (bottom). Go wider and deeper the more flexible you become.

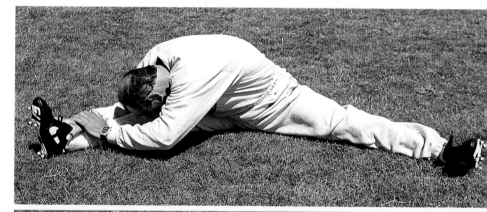

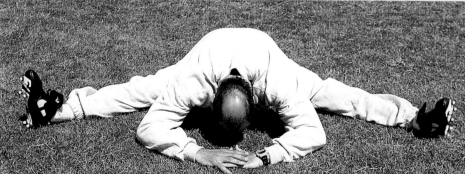

TIPS

• Use a partner wherever possible to give you a wider range of exercises
• Start off gently, gradually working your way up to a full stretch
• Know your limitations and, as with any exercise, do not over-stretch
• Always hold your positions before repeating them

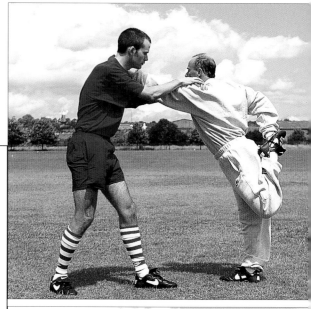

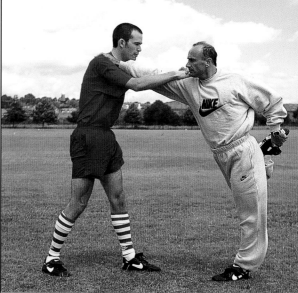

The frontal quad is a very large muscle in the thigh. It is one of the easiest to pull and one of the most difficult to heal. Muscle strains are common, particularly when players are pushing off from a standing start. The thigh can also take a number of direct blows during a game. The most common thigh complaint which footballers suffer is the 'dead leg'. Pain and tension in the thigh can also be the result of a problem elsewhere — typically this can be caused by problems in the knee or the pelvis. Good all round flexibility lessens the chance of strains, but it cannot legislate for a clumsy defender's knee going straight into your thigh. All you can do is prime your muscles by stretching properly. Two of the best thigh stretches are illustrated here.

the frontal quad

▲ ASSISTED THIGH STRETCH

This is an advanced version of a popular thigh stretch which is performed without a partner. The extra support given by your partner helps you to stretch that bit further. Do not lean too far forward, however. Try to pull your thigh all the way back so your boot touches your backside. Remember, your left arm pulls back your right leg (above) and the right arm pulls the left leg (below).

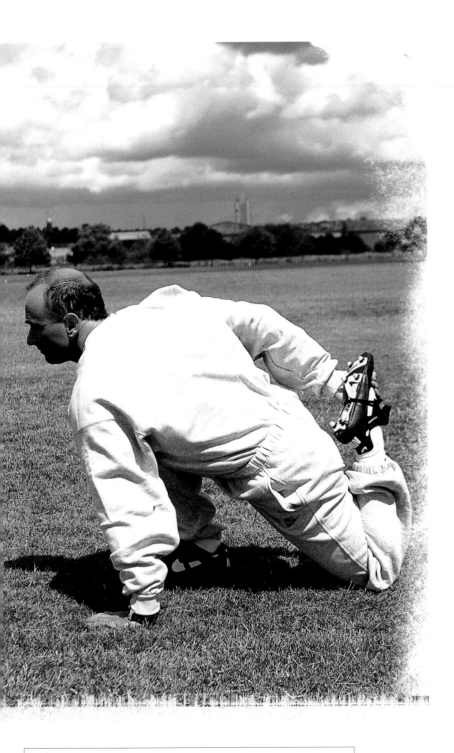

TIPS

- A version of the assisted stretch can be carried out solo, but better results are achieved with a partner
- Use your right arm to pull back your left leg and vice-versa
- Always pull your leg straight back and not at an angle when attempting these exercises
- Do not attempt advanced exercises you think might be beyond you
- Make sure you wear plenty of clothes while warming-up on a cold day, although not so much that you restrict your movement

▲ ADVANCED THIGH STRETCH

Before you carry out this exercise, always do some basic stretching first. Even then, you should only try this stretch if are a flexible person. Adopt the position as shown, using your left arm as support and your right arm to pull back your left leg. Try to keep your body at a 45-degree angle. Hold this position for ten seconds and then repeat to stretch the other leg.

the lower leg

Niggling injuries to the calf and ankle are all too common in football. However, many of these strains and pains can be prevented if you properly prepare the muscles in your lower leg.

CALF, ANKLE AND ACHILLES

The most likely muscle to be affected by cramp is the calf muscle. Most footballers know the pain of cramp in the calf only too well. The causes of cramp are the subject of much debate. Obstruction of blood/oxygen supply, salt deficiency or deficiency of other body minerals have all been blamed. All no doubt play their part, but muscle fatigue due to prolonged work is clearly a major culprit.

Development and preparation of the calf muscle will limit the chances of cramp. The calf and Achilles tendon are closely linked and often a pain in the Achilles is the result of a blow to the calf muscle. The lower leg is a very sensitive area and, therefore, requires special attention. The Achilles tendon, for example, should not be stretched too quickly or too strenuously. The ankle meanwhile is a very strong joint but, as it takes most of the force if the foot lands at an unexpected angle, the sprained ankle is the most common sports injury. 'Going over' on an ankle is very painful and results in damage to the ankle ligaments which will take about six weeks to heal. When you consider the weight the lower leg has to support and the constant pounding it takes, it becomes clear that suppleness in this area of the body is essential.

◄ CALF AND ACHILLES STRETCH

This exercise stretches the calf and Achilles. It may look awkward, but it is worth practising and getting right. Position your weight on the bent, rear leg while the front leg provides extra support. Keep your weight central and do not lean too far forward. Hold this position for 20 seconds and then repeat for the other leg.

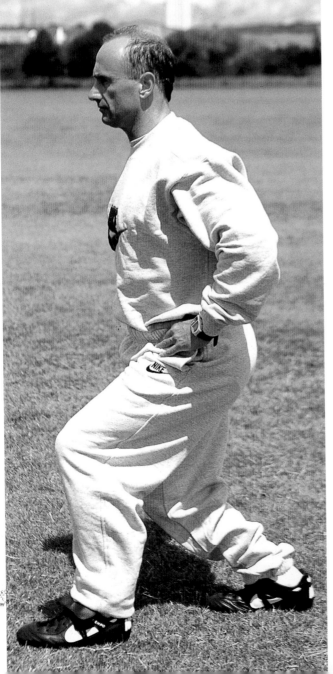

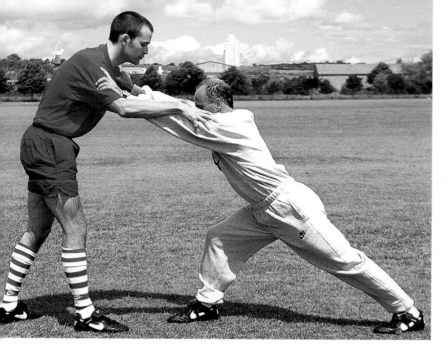

◄ ASSISTED CALF STRETCH

This exercise stretches the Achilles. Use a partner – or alternatively a wall – to push against. This helps you stretch the rear, lower leg to its maximum.

► ON ONE LEG

In addition to flexing the ankle, this exercise also works the outer and inner thigh. Use a partner for support and balance, lift your leg in the manner shown and pull the foot in towards the stomach area. Hold for ten seconds and repeat for the other leg.

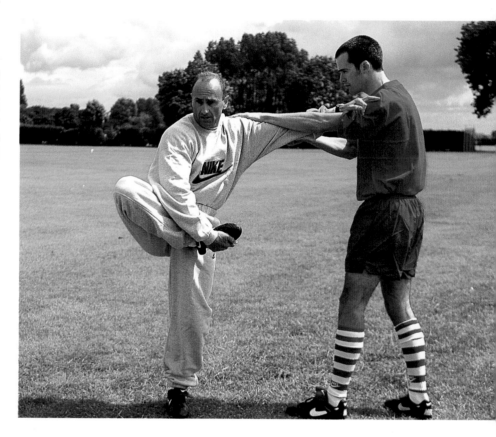

TIPS

• Treat the Achilles with care – this tendon must not be stretched quickly
• Keep both feet firmly on the ground when doing either the calf and Achilles stretch, or the assisted calf stretch
• Find your balance and hold each position for the recommended period

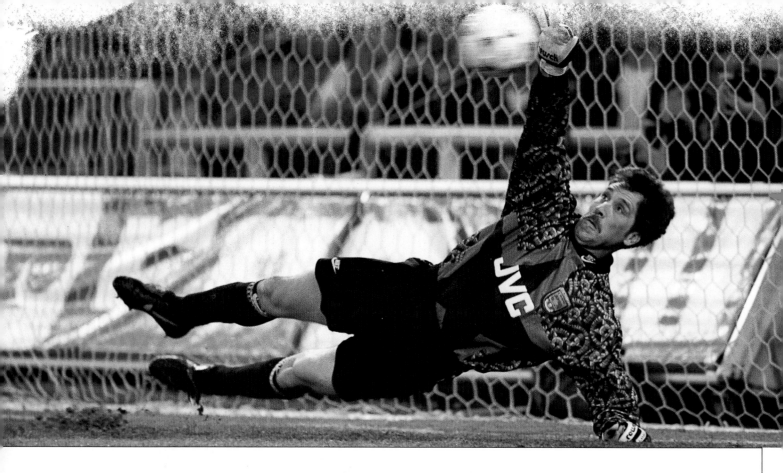

Strength training in football employs a combination of weights and specially designed anaerobic training methods to increase the physical strength of the relevant muscles and improve power and speed. This also helps improve reflexes and enables players to react quickly as things occur on the football pitch. In addition, there are benefits in rates of recovery after high-intensity work — both during training and matches. Building muscle strength can also help players avoid certain injuries which can occur at any stage of the season.

strength

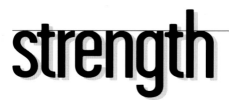

STRIKING THE BALANCE

The right level of gym work will make the body as efficient as possible for the weight you are carrying – it improves your power-to-weight ratio. However, too much weight training will mean you are carrying an excess of heavy muscle and will affect your stamina. By contrast, too little weight training will result in a loss of explosive power.

If you get it right, weight training will be particularly beneficial to players in terms of making quick, short turns and explosive bursts of speed.

Above: To be a good goalkeeper you have to be strong. You must have the strength to withstand the physical challenges of forwards and you must have the strength in your hands and arms to divert powerful shots away from your goal. Here, Arsenal keeper David Seaman shows strong hands to push away a penalty in the 1995 European Cup Winners' Cup semi-final shoot-out.

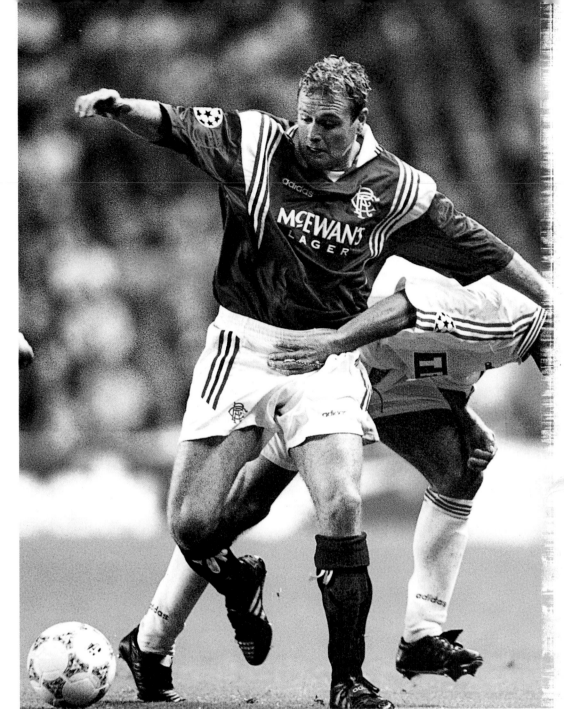

Paul Gascoigne uses his upper body strength to withstand a physical challenge while at the same time accelerating away from the challenge courtesy of the power in his legs.

WELL TRAINED MUSCLES

A correctly trained muscle uses oxygen more efficiently and, providing the muscle is strong enough, it will use less oxygen and glycogen overall. This will help aid both performance and recovery. Your body will function more efficiently, particularly during high-intensity sessions and, certainly, in the latter stages of competitive matches.

Strength increases the lactic tolerance of the muscles and, therefore, helps you to work at a high level for longer periods – reducing the possibility of the dreaded calf cramp in the process. A player with good strong muscles will also be quicker over short distances. The relationship between speed and strength is a close one.

A NOTE OF CAUTION

There is a danger that if you do too much weight training, you will become too muscular for the sport. It is about getting the balance right, carrying enough muscle to make your body efficient and achieving a good power-weight ratio. For football you need to condition your muscles, not build them.

Too much heavy muscle will effect both speed and efficiency, which is why the approach to gym work on the following pages is recommended for footballers.

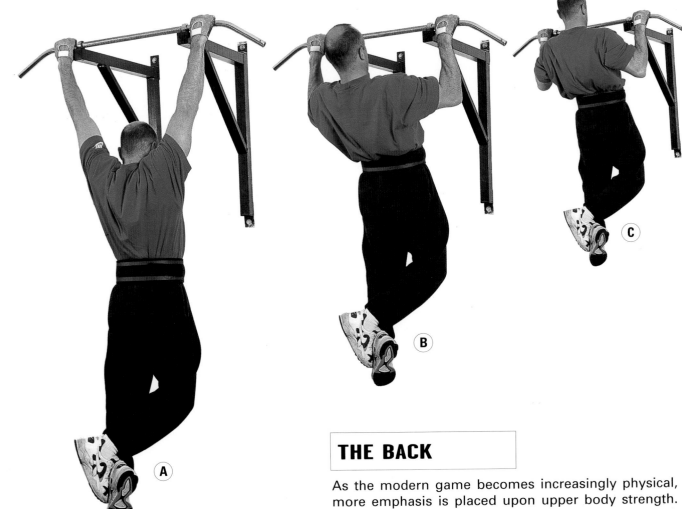

A

B

C

Work with the specialised equipment in the gym is necessary to reach the levels of strength needed for top level football.

upper body

THE BACK

As the modern game becomes increasingly physical, more emphasis is placed upon upper body strength. By working out in the gym two or three times a week your body will be better equipped to cope with football's physical demands. A strong back is important to footballers for various reasons: it helps develop power to hold off opponents and also assists with balance and agility.

The exercises demonstrated here, which are commonly called mass builders, will help you to build upper body strength. But be sensible with your weight selection – particularly where your back is concerned. Do things gradually and don't overstretch yourself. Muscle tears caused by pushing yourself too hard in the gym can put you out of action for weeks, during which time you will also lose your aerobic fitness. Allow yourself adequate rest and recovery time.

◄ CHIN UP

Pictures A, B and C show the exercise commonly known as 'chins'. This exercise is a mass builder for the upper lats and upper back muscles. It is also of secondary benefit to the biceps and forearm muscles. Start without a belt and keep your repetitions to a sensible level. As you become more competent, use weighted belts (increasing the weight as you develop) and increase the number of repeats.

Picture A shows the start position where the arms are at full stretch with the hands a little more than shoulder width apart. Note that the feet are crossed to aid balance during the exercise.

Picture B shows the mid-range position achieved by pulling the body up gently. Do not yank the bar or rush the exercise – a slow range of movement is the aim.

Picture C shows the chin, hence the name, level with the bar. Hold that position and then lower your body back down slowly. The art of coming back down is just as important as pulling yourself up.

TIPS

- Get yourself into a comfortable starting position
- Cross your feet to stop the body wobbling about during the exercise
- Do not snatch at the bar; keep the motion smooth
- When your chin reaches the bar, hold the position for a few seconds
- Lower yourself down slowly back to your starting position

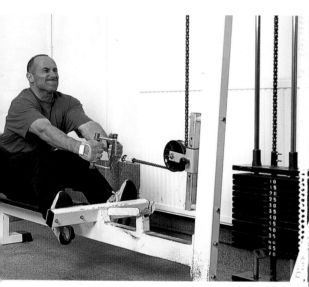

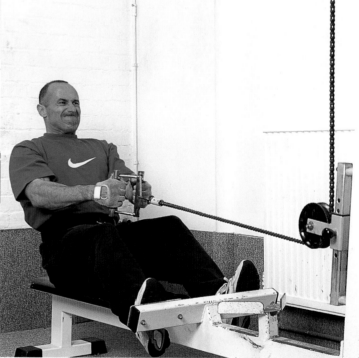

▲ LOW PULLEY ROWS

This exercise is one of the best builders of the middle area of the back, if done correctly. At the starting position your knees should be slightly bent and your arms stretched out in front of you, but do not lean too far forward. Draw the pulley towards the centre of your chest (positive action), driving your arms backwards before releasing the weight (negative action) slowly back to the original starting position.

TIPS

- Start with your knees bent, your arms stretched out in front and your back straight
- Do five sets of eight repeats with one minute rest between each
- Don't overstretch at the start – keep weights at a sensible level
- Don't release the weight too quickly – this may result in injury

the chest

It is not only your legs that need to be strong for football. A strong upper body, will enable you to hold off opponents and ride challenges.

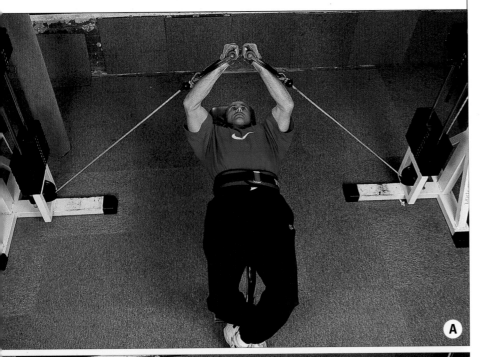

A

◄ THE CABLE FLY

The cable fly machine helps you build up the inner pectoral muscles of the chest. Pull the cable into the position shown in picture A and then lower (slowly, of course) to the position shown in picture B. At the end of each range of movement, hold the position for a few seconds before repeating. If you do not have access to a cable fly machine, you can still do this exercise using free weights by adopting the same body position and lifting and releasing the weights in the same motion.

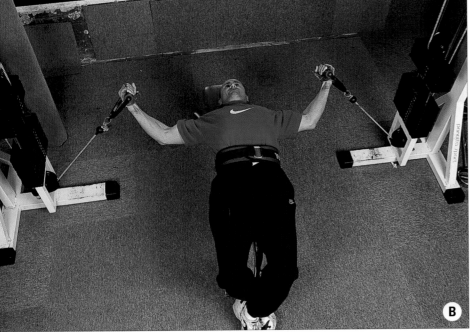

B

TIPS

- Do the full range of motion – don't cheat yourself
- Pull the cable above your head
- Do not release the weight too quickly
- Use free weights if necessary, but take great care and don't be tempted to over-stretch yourself

Using a partner to assist you, you can increase the weights you use. He will also help you achieve a few extra repeats.

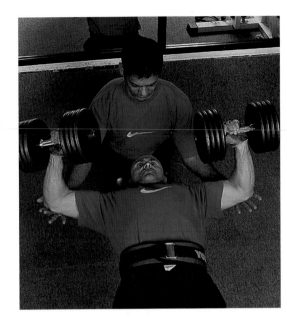

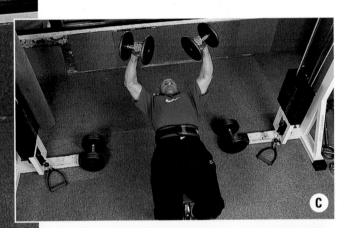

C

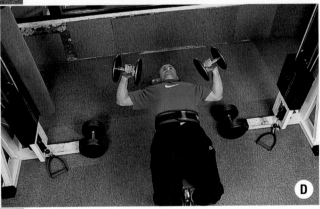

D

◄ THE DUMB BELL PRESS

Using a bench positioned at a 45-degree angle, raise the dumb bells above the chest and back to the starting position as in the illustration. This exercise can also be done on a flat bench (Pictures C and D) to build up the mid and lower area of the pectorals.

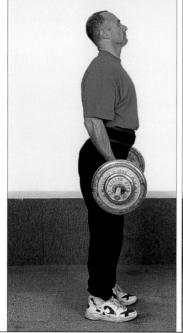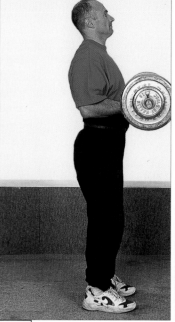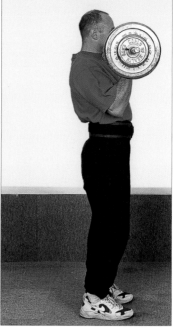

arms

You might think that unless you are a goalkeeper — or perhaps the team's long throw expert — that strong arms are not important. But this is not the case. You should ideally work your whole body. Devise a balanced work-out and try not to miss out any part of your body.

▲ STRAIGHT BAR BELL CURVE

Start this exercise with your body upright and the weight resting on your thigh. Your feet should be about 12 inches apart.

Using the natural curve your arms make as you raise the weights, lift the bar to the mid-way position as shown in Picture B. Keep your elbows tucked into the body to maintain the weight on the biceps.

Complete the curve so that the weight is almost resting on your chest and hold that position. Lower the weight slowly to the starting position and repeat this eight times. Do five sets of eight repeats with a minute's rest in between each one.

TIPS

- Hold the bar with your palms facing upwards
- Keep your back (supported by a belt) straight at all times
- Keep your elbows tucked into your side
- The motion should be smooth – do not swing the weight around
- Lower the weight slowly to work the forearms
- Add weights gradually as you develop

The legs are the most important part of a footballer's equipment. The better you look after them the less likely you are to pick up an injury. Running, playing and everyday training keeps the legs in good shape and prepares you for 90 minutes of action. But by working both the upper and lower leg – exercising the joints and developing the muscles – you can make your body a more effective machine and one which is fully equipped to cope with the rigours of modern football.

Strong legs are important to all players, but it is important not to build too much heavy muscle as this can have an adverse effect on performance.

Get the balance right between the number of repetitions you do and the weight you are lifting. There are times for high reps but there are also times to work with heavier weights to bring more of the fibres in the relevant muscles into play. Increase the weights gradually and in doing so increase the ability of the muscle to work at a better capacity. This approach will have positive benefits on the field of play. A simple rule is reduce the weights for maximum reps; increase the weight for reduced reps. Footballers should not try to build too much muscle because this will be only be counterbalanced by their essential aerobic training.

TIPS

• Weight training machines should only be used after proper instruction from a qualified trainer
• Take your time when using machines; do not be hurried by other people who wish to use your machine

legs

The legs must clearly be the most important limbs for a footballer — they are at work for 90 minutes non-stop during a game, whether you are kicking, running or just standing still. They need the right exercise and care, and their strength must be built up without an excess of muscle.

THE HACK SQUAT

This exercise helps to build the front quad area – one of the most important areas of the leg for kicking.

Starting in the squat position, with your hands holding the bars either side of the machine for extra leverage (picture A), push your weight downwards until your body is fully upright but with your feet flat on the metal plate (picture B). Slowly bend your knees to the starting position and repeat.

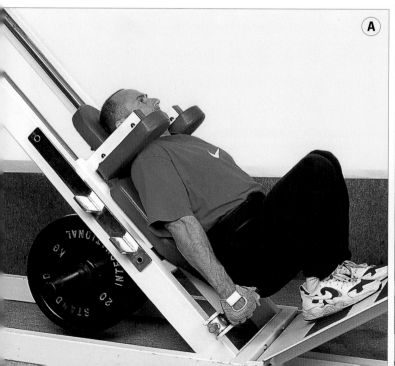

(A)

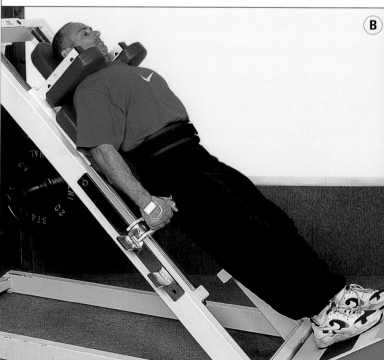

(B)

legs

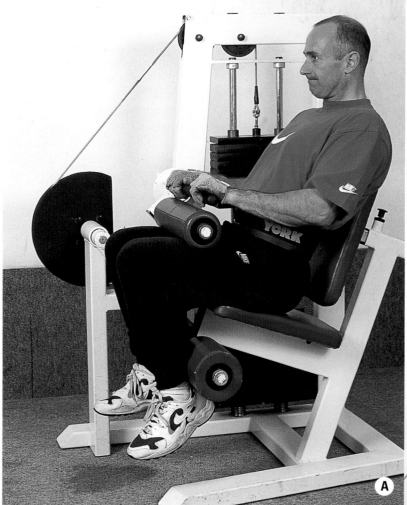

WORKING YOUR THIGHS

Each area of the leg needs a different approach. When working on the thigh, it is important to do a lot of repetitions using low weights before moving on.

THE HAMSTRING CURL

Adopt the position illustrated and bend the legs to bring the weight into the position in picture A. Release the weight slowly back to the starting position with the legs straight out in front of you (picture B). This exercise strengthens the rear leg bicep which helps improve acceleration.

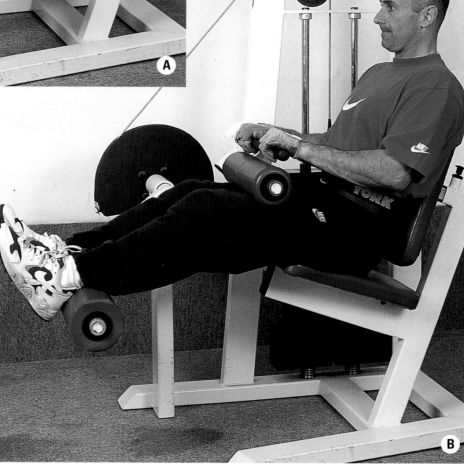

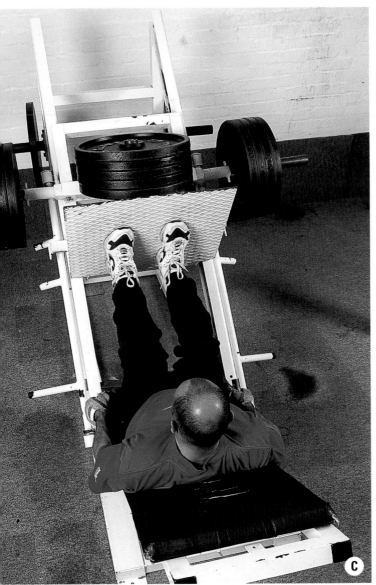

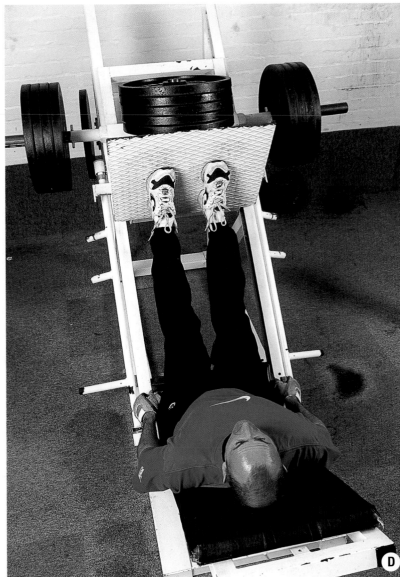

THE LEG PRESS

This exercise builds the larger part of the quad (thigh) muscle.

Picture C
With both the weight machine and the bench at 45 degrees, position yourself with your legs bent almost to your chest and your feet flat against the metal plate.

Picture D
Extend your legs until they are at full stretch and hold the position with your legs locked. The movement should be smooth yet with enough force to work your legs. Lower the weight slowly back to the starting position and repeat eight times.

TIPS

• Keep your back flat against the padded bench and wear a belt for support
• Keep your hands by your side Extend your legs smoothly but powerfully
• Lower the weights slowly in order to maximise the negative movement

anaerobic training

The term anaerobic means 'without air' and is used to describe exercise which is intense, such as sprinting or weight training. It is inefficient, compared to aerobic activity, and requires you to work your heart very hard. Anaerobic activity cannot be sustained for long periods.

Football is a game which requires both aerobic and anaerobic fitness. For parts of a game, you will work anaerobically – most commonly this will come in the form of short sprints, during which you will build up an oxygen debt and lactic acid in your muscles. These periods are followed by longer spells of jogging and walking. However, at any time during a game you must be ready to enter oxygen debt and go anaerobic.

In order to sustain these periods of exertion, you must build up your tolerance to anaerobic exercise by working it into your training schedule. In this way, your body will be better prepared to adapt and cope with high-intensity exercise and lactate pressure. You will also reduce your recovery time...not to mention your desire to stand with your hands on hips, gasping for air after making a 30m run. If you are going to compete for 90 minutes, you have to expose yourself to anaerobic exercise in your training.

Anaerobic training is always hard work. These players are wearing specially designed parachutes attached to their backs while sprinting in short bursts. The extra resistance helps build both their strength and speed.

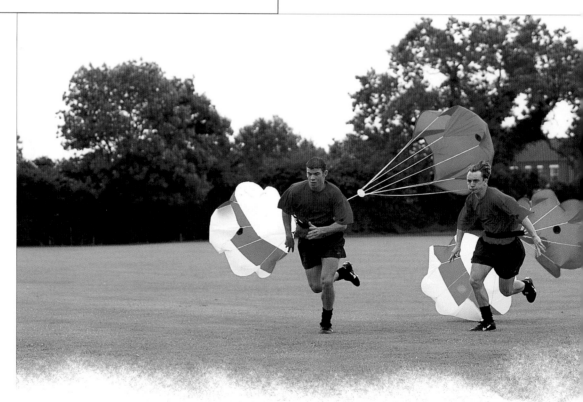

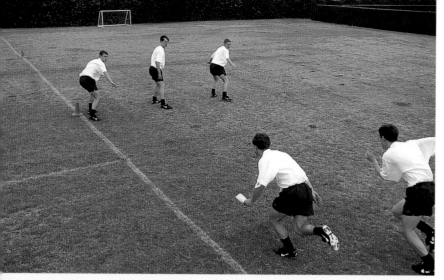

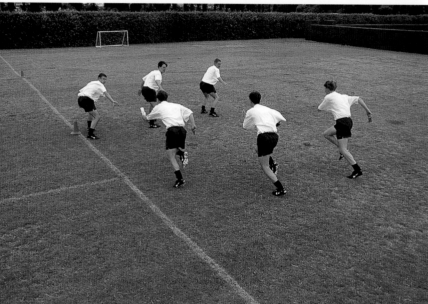

SPRINT TRAINING

Short-burst training will improve your anaerobic fitness. Sprints of between five and ten seconds, followed by a walk back to the starting point and repeating the sprint are ideal. Players should work to their maximum capacity for these short periods. This sort of work helps increase your lactate threshold.

The danger with anaerobic training is that there is a high risk of injury because you are pushing yourself so hard. For this reason, you should not do this type of exercise too often. Use it occasionally, perhaps only once every 2–3 weeks, in order to supplement your regular training programme.

If your body can cope with this sort of high-intensity work-out, you have a better chance of making that 50m surge in the last few minutes of a game.

Shuttle runs are an excellent form of sprint training. Short bursts of sprinting are followed by periods of recovery before the run is repeated.

The ability to make a quick run at the end of a tiring game is a major asset to any player. Training exercises aimed at building this type of speed endurance require the player to work against resistance. Here the coach is holding the player back by a tape worn across his midrift. Other speed endurance exercises employ weighted jackets to get players working hard.

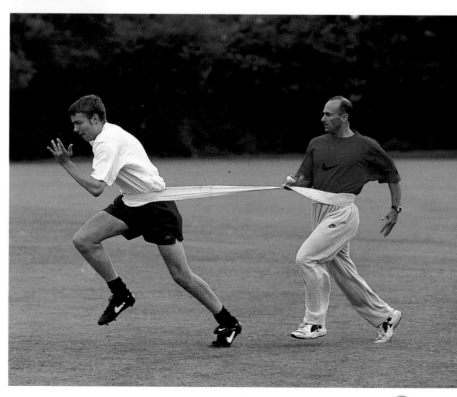

JARGON BUSTER

• Anaerobic training involves short, quick bursts – between 5 and 7 seconds. Sprint up, walk back and sprint again
• Aerobic training involves longer runs – anything over 15 seconds. You run and then warm-down

plymetrics

Plymetrics is not about speed over distance, although it can improve this, it is about that initial burst from the blocks.

FIRST OUT OF THE BLOCKS

Plymetric training helps develop explosive power within the muscles and there are various ways of achieving this. The most common ways use hurdles, benches and hoops for hopping, jumping and side-stepping with an explosive action. This type of exercise stimulates the mytatic reflex (the sort of reaction you get when someone touches your arm with a recently extinguished match).

By improving this aspect of your fitness, you can turn more quickly and get away from opponents. It gives you a little extra explosive pace which can make a great difference. Even if you are not blessed with great speed, by improving your plymetric fitness, you will be able to compete with the fastest player over that all-important first yard.

This sort of training also improves agility and co-ordination, thus enabling you to change direction quickly – a major benefit in the modern game.

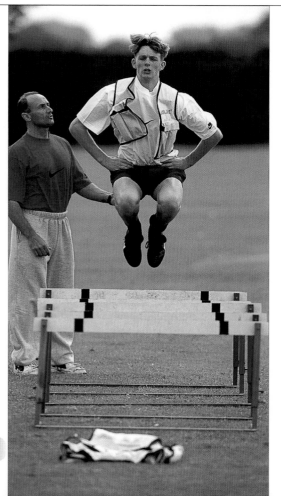
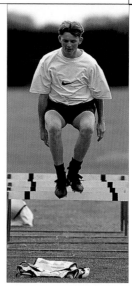
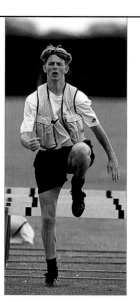
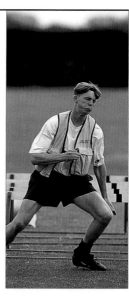

A great deal of plymetric training uses hurdles to help sharpen reactions within the muscles. This exercise requires players to put on a weighted jacket, before jumping on the spot (with knees up high and hands on hips as shown) five times. The player then removes the weighted jacket, jumps the five hurdles, puts on the weighted jacket once more, runs on the spot for 10 seconds and then turns sharply and sprints back to the starting position. This exercise improves not only plymetric fitness, but also speed and speed endurance.

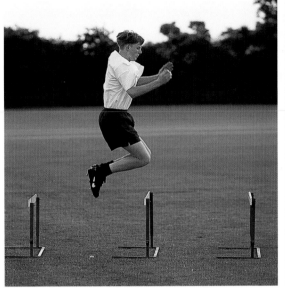

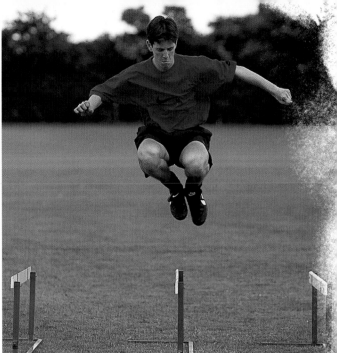

Jumping over hurdles is a great way to improve plymetric fitness. This type of training should only be used occasionally and for short periods however. Try to vary the exercises – jumping hurdles from side to side (as shown right) for example.

SAFETY FIRST

Plymetric training must be carried out on a soft surface. There is a big shock or impact factor involved in this kind of explosive training and it is important to take precautions against injury (jarring of the knee, twisting of the ankle, etc.). Ideally you should use either grass, or a training mat in a gym. It is also essential to wear shoes that offer both support and cushioning.

It is equally important when working in this way to be thoroughly warmed up beforehand – just as you would before taking part in a game itself. Training sessions which involve this kind of explosive intensity should last no more than 20 minutes and should be carried out no more than twice a week. Any more than this and you are making excessive demands of your body and increasing the risk of injury. Train hard, but train sensibly – and allow yourself adequate recovery time in between.

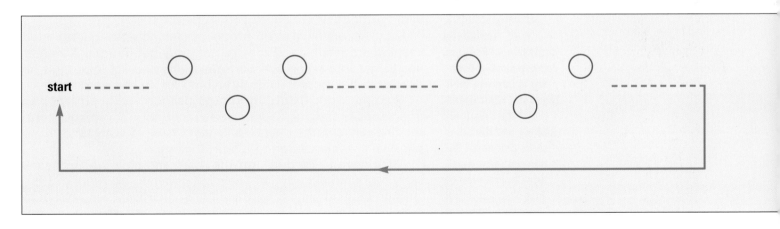

○ – hoop

- - - – short quick steps

—— – sprint to start

If you don't have any hurdles with which to train, an alternative plymetric exercise can be performed with just six hoops. Each player starts with three short steps, before hopping on one foot in each of the three hoops. They then move to the next set of hoops via three short steps, hop in each hoop, move on to the end by three short steps and then sprint to the start.

goalkeeper fitness

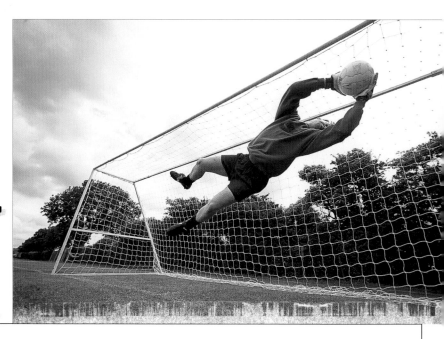

Goalkeepers are so often the forgotten men when it comes to training, but their fitness is just as important as the fitness of any of the outfield players.

Traditionally, goalkeeper training involved hitting a few crosses and shots at the keeper after he'd spent an hour or so running around a field. Nowadays professional keepers receive special training to improve their reactions, their speed off the line, their kicking and the other skills that make the difference between three points won or lost. This approach should be adopted at all levels of the game.

Goalkeeper training varies dramatically from that of outfield players, although the same fitness principles still apply. In particular, keepers need to do more explosive training and jumping, rather than running and speed work. They have to become more agile and develop quicker reflexes, both with and without the ball. To this end, keepers should do a lot of plymetric work with hurdles and weight jackets in their training.

Goalkeepers have to do a lot of stretching work too. All good keepers are flexible – if they're not, they get injured. A keeper has to get into some awkward positions and it's important he doesn't pull a muscle while stretching for an awkward ball.

Strength work in the gym should also form an important part of a keeper's training. Upper body strength is a valuable commodity between the posts, as keepers have to withstand many physical challenges during a typical game.

They have to be quick off the mark and alert which means carrying minimal body fat. They will generally be more muscular than outfield players, particularly in their legs, which have to supply the power and spring to reach high balls. Plymetric jump training is used to improve goalkeepers' spring.

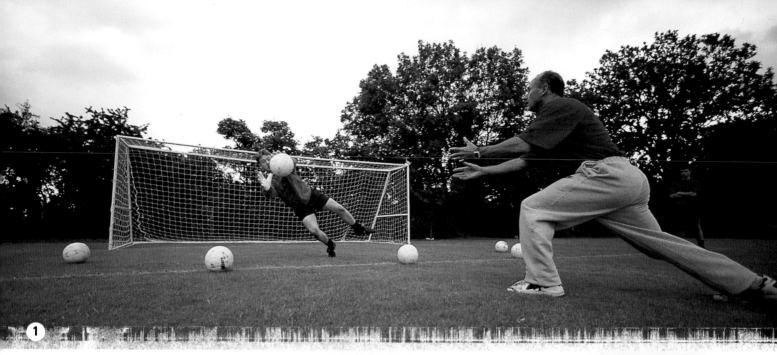

DIET AND PLAYING IN GOAL

Goalkeepers do not do as much aerobic activity as outfield players and for this reason, they must take great care about what they eat. An hour and a half between the posts will not burn off a portion of fish and chips or an extra slice of chocolate cake. It is essential that keepers stay trim; the more weight they are carrying the more they have got to work to spring and jump. Power-weight ratios are just as important to keepers as they are to outfield players. A good healthy diet with a large proportion of carbohydrate will help prevent weight gain and sluggish goalkeeping.

A BALANCED ROUTINE

Ideally, keepers should divide their training time between the training ground and the gym. Time in the gym should be spent building up their body strength and doing springing work off the benches and squats. Speed and strength are closely related. If a keeper works hard on his strength, he will be quick off his line.

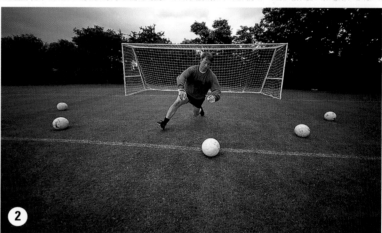

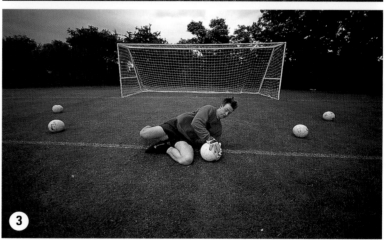

This exercise helps to improve both reactions and speed off the line. Five balls are spaced in an arc around the six yard box and each ball is numbered. The coach then stands on the penalty spot and throws balls at the keeper to save. At any point during the exercise (and without warning) the coach shouts out a number and the keeper must dive onto the corresponding ball. The coach resumes throwing balls from the penalty spot immediately.

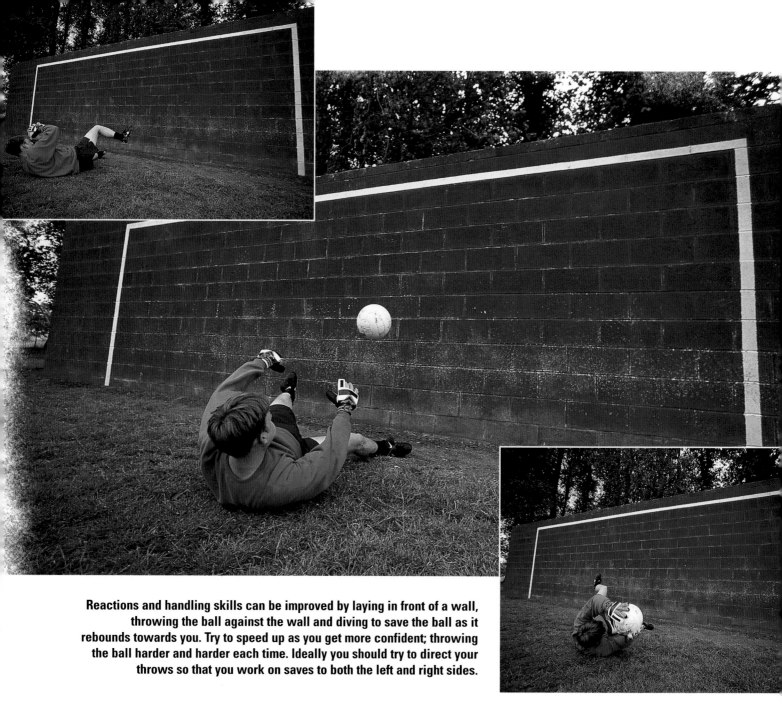

Reactions and handling skills can be improved by laying in front of a wall, throwing the ball against the wall and diving to save the ball as it rebounds towards you. Try to speed up as you get more confident; throwing the ball harder and harder each time. Ideally you should try to direct your throws so that you work on saves to both the left and right sides.

WARM-UP

A keeper's warm-up should be slightly different to that of an outfield player. Greater emphasis is placed on stretching – particularly the arms and upper body. It is imperative to warm-up properly, especially in the winter when strains can occur if the muscles aren't prepared properly. By the same token, if you are lucky enough to play for a team where you have nothing to do for long periods, you should stretch throughout the game. However keep an eye on what's going on a the other end!

THE MENTAL GAME

At professional level, keepers work with a specific goalkeeper coach for several days a week. The coach will work on the player's handling, but will also try and build confidence. If a keeper loses his confidence, the whole team are in trouble, so it is important that training sessions do not demoralise goalkeepers. Concentration is another essential element in a keeper's game, but the only way to improve this is to play plenty of practice matches.

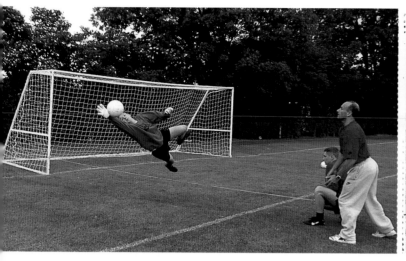
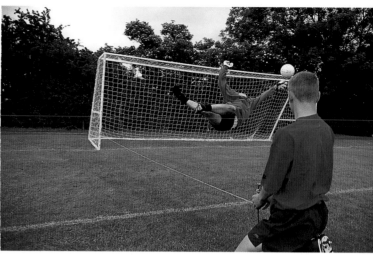

The art of goalkeeping is not just about getting your hands to the ball, it's about getting enough power in your save to protect your goal. The exercise shown above helps develop the keeper's spring and push, by forcing him to dive over a rope (held by the player kneeling down). The coach throws the ball to one side of the rope and then, before the keeper has had time to recover properly, throws one to the other side. This improves the keepers reactions.

Note: The rope should always be held low down and must be held relaxed enough to avoid injury to the keeper if he catches himself on it.

PLYMETRICS ON BENCHES

Quick reactions are essential to goalkeepers, so plymetric exercises form an important part of their training. The simple, but effective, exercise illustrated left, involves two benches laid side by side. Each player hops from foot to foot in a zig-zag pattern across the two benches.

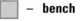 – bench

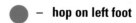 – hop on left foot

– hop on right foot

TIP

• A popular routine used by top keepers is to stand in a circle of discs, each of which has a different number. The coach calls out a number and the keeper has to run to that disc, dive on it, run back to the centre of the circle and then go again

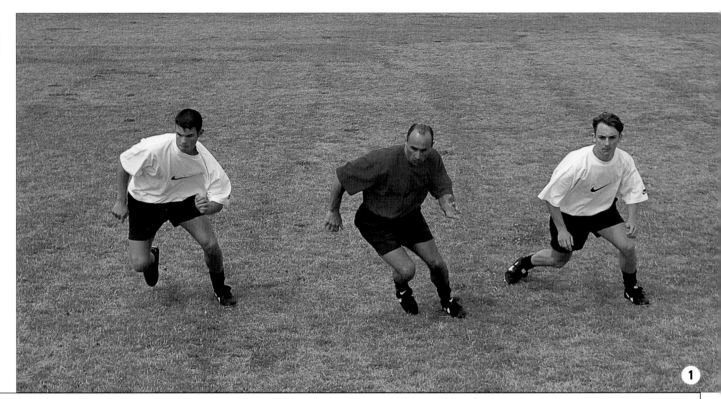

All footballers, whatever their position, need a certain level of base fitness. But once this is achieved, each player must concentrate on improving specific areas of their fitness. The biggest single factor dictating the areas a player should concentrate upon is his position within the team. For example, a centre-forward must develop pace and strength whereas a midfielder must work more on stamina. The game makes different demands on every player and you must be prepared to meet those demands.

training for outfield players

DEFENDERS

It's a myth that defenders don't have to be fit. In the past, there may have been some truth in this, but nowadays defenders are expected to join in attacks, support their midfielders and get back to do their own job. Full-backs and wing-backs, in particular, need a great deal of stamina. This role requires you to cover a great deal of ground. In some systems you will be expected to cover the whole flank – operating as a winger when you're attacking and tracking back and covering like an orthodox defender.

At professional level, full-backs and wing-backs would use specially designed parachutes to build up their stamina and work rate. These parachutes are attached to the players and offer a solid resistance to their legs which makes them stronger and quicker to react. Full-backs would wear them for repeated runs of 50 yards. Similar running exercises are carried out while wearing weighted jackets – these jackets make the player carry an extra 10% of his body weight. This sort of training should only be introduced into the training session every 4-6 weeks.

If you can't get hold of specialist items like weight jackets and parachutes, an ordinary jacket with weight in the pockets, or a car tyre attached to a belt via a rope can work just as well.

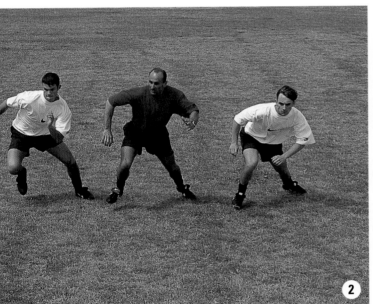

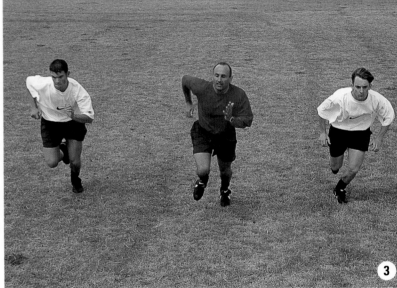

Pictures 1–3 illustrate a simple exercise which helps to improve speed, reaction and acceleration. The coach (in red) directs the players with a shout to move left (pic 1) via an exaggerated step, then move right (pic 2) via a similar step and then finally to accelerate straight ahead (pic 3). This exercise can be repeated several times, or alternatively incorporated into a longer run.

YOUNG OR OLD

Power training with weight jackets and parachutes is extremely strenuous and so you must consider the age of the players you are working with. Do not ask a 32-year-old to produce the same results as a 22-year-old. Older players must be allowed greater time for recovery, before the next exertion, than their younger team-mates.

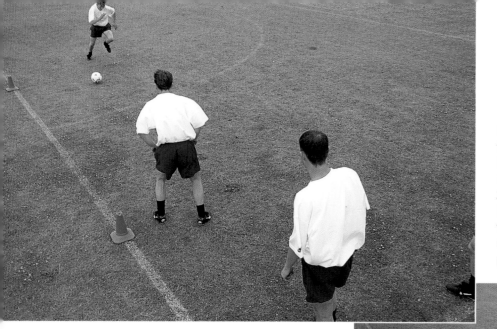

Some of the best fitness exercises incorporate the ball as well, and in this way they help to improve technique at the same time. This exercise requires each player to dribble the ball to a 20-metre mark, turn and run back with the ball, before releasing a 10-metre pass to a team-mate who receives the ball and sets out on the same run. The exercise is repeated after a recovery period while the team-mate completes his run.

CENTRAL DEFENDERS

Training for full-backs is very similar to midfielders. Central defenders need different exercises to hone their fitness for their job on the field. In recent years the role of the central defender has become more demanding, as changes to the back-pass rule have required players to work around 10% harder than they did under the old regulations. Pace has also become more important – as strikers get quicker, defenders must speed up to keep up. To develop the pace of central defenders the same sort of speed endurance work with parachutes used for full-backs is recommended. This helps improve their speed over short distances, which is particularly valuable to central defenders who are often faced with situations where they have to turn and run back towards their own goal to track a lively striker.

The weighted jacket is also useful to help develop a central defender's spring. If a player can become accustomed to jumping with a heavy weighted jacket in training sessions, he will find aerial challenges easy on a match day. This training will also improve players' overall fitness and enable them to last longer during a game.

Body strength is also important to central defenders. It is important for them to have enough power to hold players off, particularly the big, bustling centre-forwards who are going to present a physical and aerobic test.

Gym work is therefore important for central defenders.

PARACHUTE TRAINING

Specially designed parachutes have been employed for some time in Italian football training. They are used to develop speed with a minimum risk of injury. Parachutes can also help players to develop the ability to change direction quickly – something all players have to do from time to time.

For example, if a gust of wind catches the chute it throws the player off balance – as if he has been knocked by another player – and he has to re-adjust and change his direction.

If they are used correctly, parachutes can improve both strength and explosive pace and can be used to get players back to full fitness after injury. This type of training employs many of the fibres in the leg muscles and improves a player's power. The parachutes also provide valuable variety in football training and keep players interested in the session.

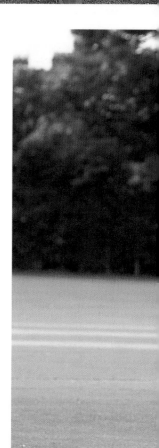

FORWARDS

Forwards have to be fitter nowadays because they must close defenders down rather than simply hold a central position. Strikers who play up front on their own have to be supremely fit, as they must cover a huge amount of ground. To develop this kind of stamina you'll need to follow a programme of running (see page 18). Whatever system your team plays, you will need to have good explosive power and acceleration to play up front. Resistance training (i.e. parachute work) is the best way to develop this type of speed. Strength, too, is important to a front man so make sure you follow a sensible programme of training in a gym (see pages 34–43).

MIDFIELD

Midfield players need to develop a high level of stamina. They will be expected to make runs, cover and tackle back for the whole of the game. The only way to prepare for this kind of exertion is to do plenty of running in training (see page 18). Defensive midfielders, who are going to be involved in aerial challenges and tackles more than attacking runs, should take elements of their training from that recommended for defenders. Similarly, attacking midfielders should concentrate on stamina plus elements from the forwards' programme (see right). Plymetric training is particularly valuable for all midfielders as in the middle of the field you will have to react quickly as the ball is played through congested areas and as attack changes to defence.

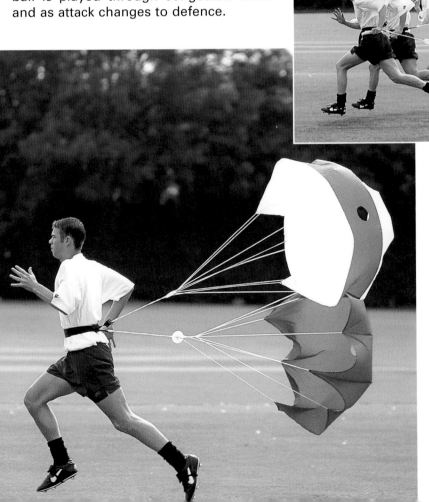

Specially designed parachutes are used in professional football training to develop speed and reaction. Traditionally this type of running-resistance has been provided by weight jackets or by tyres pulled on a rope attached to a player's belt. The parachutes have the advantage over the older methods, because they change direction with the wind, thus forcing players to react quickly and adjust their run.

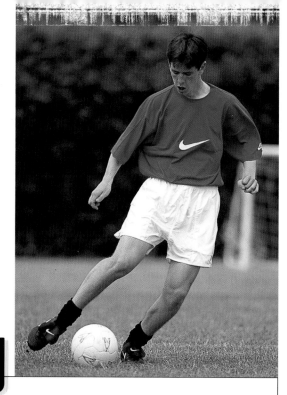

high-intensity training

The aim of high-intensity training is to keep the heart rate high and the body working at a level which is similar to that of a match situation. A player will work in excess of 75% of his maximum level during a match. High-intensity training should reflect this — albeit for shorter periods. In some cases, training should be more physically demanding than a match, with players working at between 75% and 95% of their maximum output. By pushing themselves over and above what they'd expect to do in a match, those last gruelling 15 minutes of a game won't be so bad.

WARM-UP

As with any type of football training, it is important to carry out a proper warm-up before beginning a high-intensity session. If you are planning a high-intensity training session, then a high-intensity warm-up should precede it. The body will be warm, the muscles prepared and the heart rate reaching a level needed for the sort of hard work which follows. A high-intensity session will replicate the exertions of a proper match, so your wam-up should be the same as your match preparation.

HARD BUT NOT TOO HARD

The majority of high-intensity training takes the form of small-sided games, although exercises can be done without the ball. Either way, the aim is to keep the body working at a high heart rate and a high state of lactate. However, it's not about pushing yourself until you drop. Running shuttles until you collapse through exhaustion is not the way ahead. All you are doing is knocking your legs out. Yes, the idea is to push yourself, but not kill yourself.

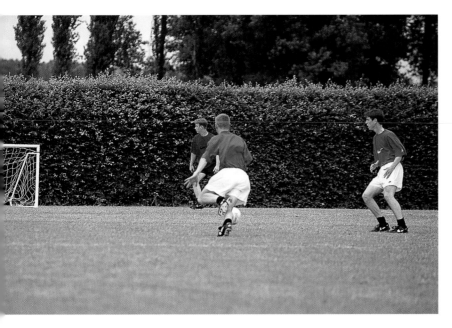

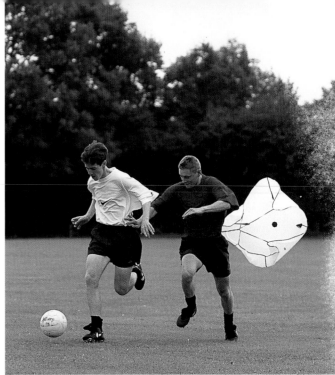

HIGH-INTENSITY SESSION

An ideal session would comprise some short sprint work (short runs with six repeats) but, in the main, would be built around various small-sided games. An example of this is a four v four practice match on a small pitch with eight other players standing around the pitch, acting as a wall to keep the ball in play and keep the intensity as high as possible.

These games last anything between 4–8 minutes. At the end of this period, the players rotate with those standing on the outside of the pitch. In total, the session should last no longer than 45 minutes.

Left: Small-sided games are an excellent and enjoyable form of high-intensity training. Try to make sure that all players are working hard during the session and get the ball into play quickly when it goes outside the playing area.

Above: If a coach wants to work particular players very hard during a high-intensity session, he can give them extra resistance, for example a parachute or a weighted jacket.

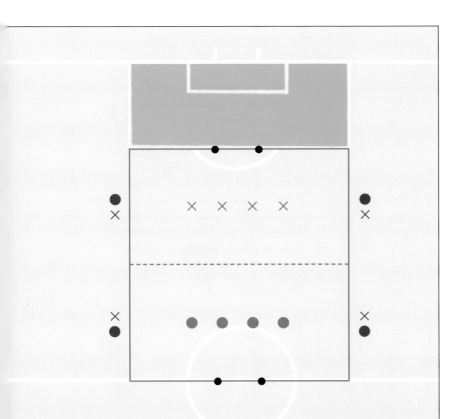

●	–	goalpost
✕	–	team A
●	–	team B
- -	–	shooting line
●✕	–	players resting from teams C+D. Their job is to get the ball back into the playzone quickly

This high-intensity four v four game uses a small area of pitch with resting players standing around the playing area ready to get the ball back into play should it go 'dead'. There are no goalkeepers, but shooting is only allowed within a marked area. After five minutes the players on the outside swap with those in the playzone.

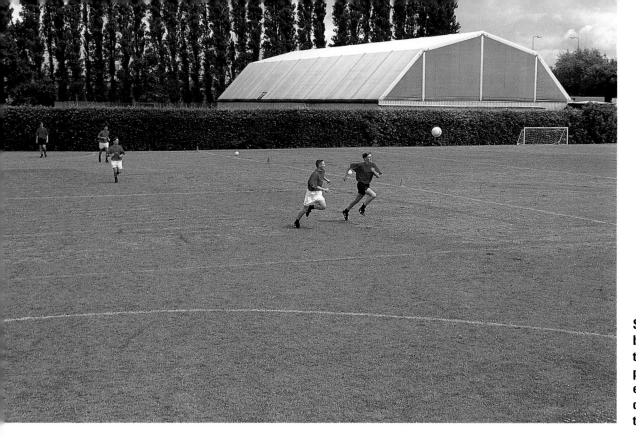

Small sided games bring out the competitive side in most players. They are an excellent way of developing both technique and fitness.

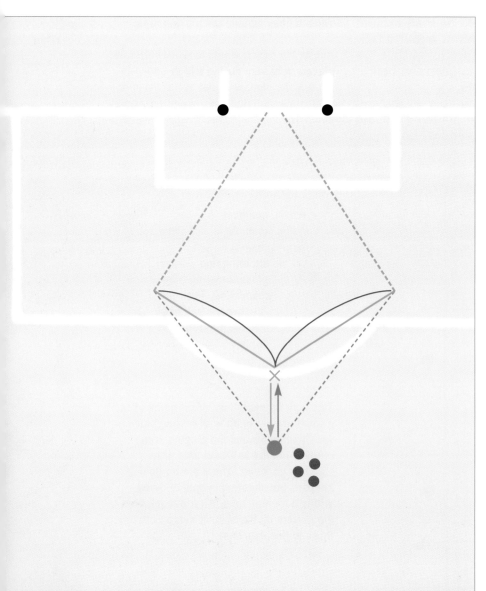

●	–	footballs
—	–	player's return run
—	–	player's sprint
- -	–	player's shot
- -	–	server's pass
●	–	server
●	–	goal
✕	–	player

Left: This high-intensity exercise is intended to develop the reactions and finishing of all outfield players, but particularly forwards. The server and player exchange short passes, before (without warning) the server plays a ball into space which the player must turn and sprint onto, before hitting a shot on goal. The player must then run immediately back to his mark.

high-intensity training continued

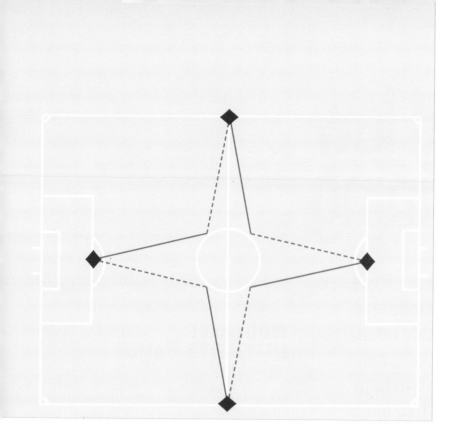

RECOVERY

It is essential to give the body enough time to recover between high-intensity exercises or games. If you are working without the ball, for example, you should train for 8–12 minutes and then allow 2–3 minutes for rest before starting work again. This process can be continued for about an hour – though no longer.

High-intensity training is an excellent way for older players to maintain their fitness. However, it is important to take an extended recovery period in between exercises.

It is imperative that high-intensity sessions contain enough time for players to recover. Without recovery time, fitness will be eroded rather than developed. As a rough guide, you should allow three minutes of rest for every 10 minutes of exertion.

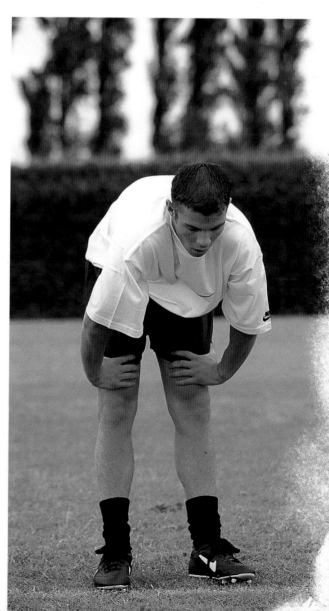

moderate and low intensity training

For training after a game or after a high-intensity work-out, a moderate-intensity session is ideal. The body needs time to recover from a hard work-out, and I would never recommend doing two high-intensity sessions back-to-back. This leads to over-tiredness and risks of muscle strains and all sorts of other injuries.

A moderate session, as the name implies, involves a reasonable work-out but does not push the body to the sort of levels of exertion involved in a high-intensity session. These sessions are purely aerobic; players are not required to work their hearts hard or go into oxygen debt. Because of the slower pace of these sessions, it is easy to introduce the ball into exercises and so develop technique as well as fitness.

MODERATE INTENSITY GAMES

A typical moderate-intensity session would begin with a warm-up and stretch – this would not need to be as vigorous as the high-intensity warm-up, as the pulse will not be taken to such a high level during the session. When warm, players would divide into teams and prepare for a small-sided game. There are many variations of low-intensity small-sided games, but all have one aim…to restrict the movement and pace of the game. This can be achieved by playing on a larger pitch, but marking the playing area into zones which players cannot move from. Alternatively, players can be restricted to three touches in certain areas and free football in others which can be coupled with restrictions being placed upon players going into certain areas of the pitch in an effort to prevent them over-stretching themselves. As with the high-intensity games, sessions should last around 45 minutes. Players should not exert themselves too much during these games, although you can back the game up with some moderate-intensity running.

Other examples of moderate games include head tennis or possesion games involving a handful of players in a circle.

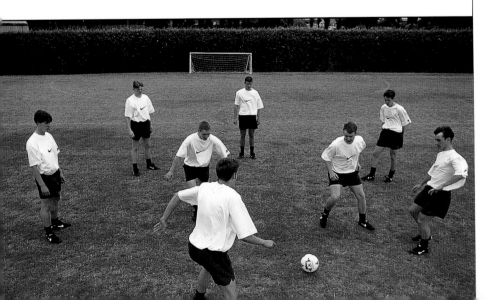

A tight passing circle with two players trying to intercept is an enjoyable low-intensity exercise which helps to develop technique as well.

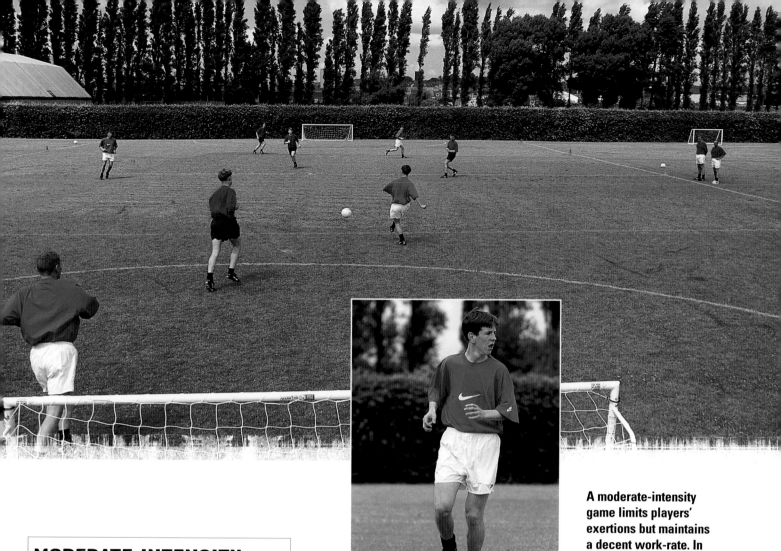

A moderate-intensity game limits players' exertions but maintains a decent work-rate. In the main picture, the ball is played through the walk zone.

MODERATE-INTENSITY TWO-TOUCH GAME

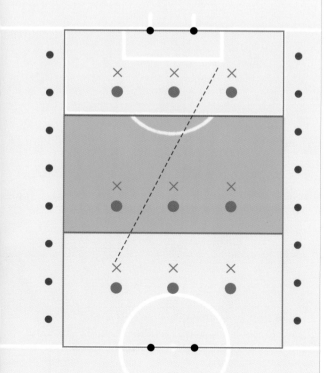

- ▨ — walk zone, no tackling
- ● — goalpost
- ✕ — team A
- ● — team B
- – – — pass
- ● — footballs

In the moderate-intensity game, players are restricted to particular areas to limit their exertion and in the central third of the pitch, tackling is not allowed. Passes are allowed between any zones (as illustrated) and balls are ready on the sidelines to keep the game running.

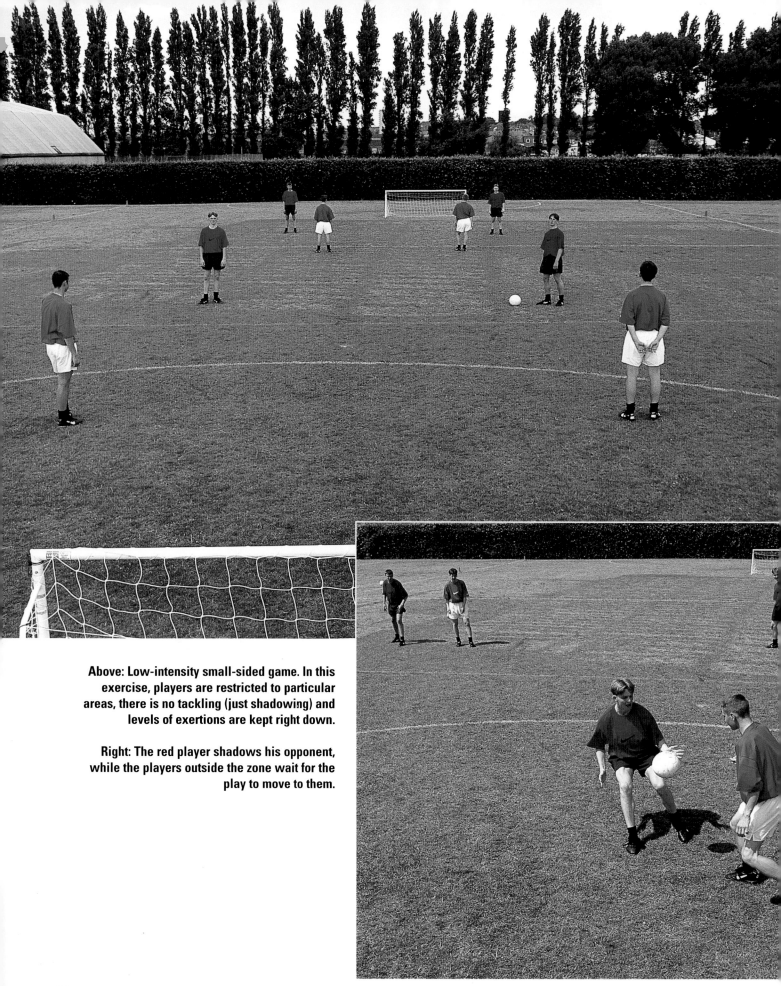

Above: Low-intensity small-sided game. In this exercise, players are restricted to particular areas, there is no tackling (just shadowing) and levels of exertions are kept right down.

Right: The red player shadows his opponent, while the players outside the zone wait for the play to move to them.

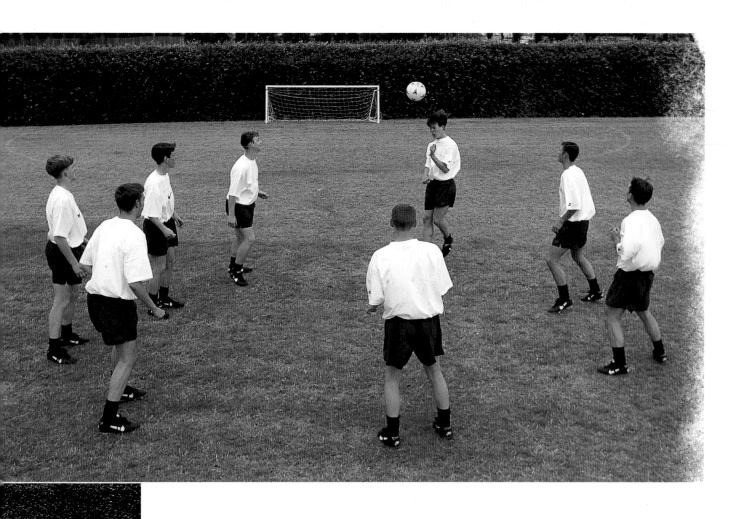

LOW-INTENSITY GAMES

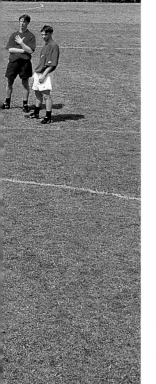

Low-intensity sessions usually involve squaring off an area of the training field, dividing it up into areas from which players are not allowed to move and playing a small-sided game. Players cannot travel – or pass the ball in certain cases – from zone to zone. In this way, the game is played at little more than a jogging pace.

This type of game can be used to help to lower the intensity of the work gradually after a strenuous session. In doing so, it helps the recovery process.

Low-intensity games based around full-sized games are also used prior to a game. These games are usually punctuated by discussions about tactics and set plays.

Above: Head tennis is a good form of low-intensity training. The emphasis is on developing technique, but it still makes players concentrate and work a little too.

warm-up

Warm-up is not just something for the pros. Whatever level you play the game at, you owe it to yourself and your team-mates to prepare your body properly for the exertions to come.

STRETCH YOUR MUSCLES

A good warm-up will gradually increase the blood flow in your body, raise the temperature of the muscles and improve their flexibility. Muscle temperature reaches a suitable level after about ten minutes, which is why it is recommended that the warm-up period should last between 10 and 15 minutes and certainly no longer than 20. In effect, your warm-up will get your body into an aerobic state to withstand strenuous, physical exercise. If you try to warm-up during the fast and frantic opening 15 minutes of a game, you will place a tremendous strain on your muscles. Injuries occur when the muscles have not been sufficiently warmed up. A cold muscle is more rigid and a sudden or rapid movement means it is unable to respond quickly enough and can tear.

'When a muscle is raised in temperature, its performance and flexibility are enhanced by around 20%.'

THE BENEFITS OF WARM-UP

Do not underestimate the importance of warming-up before training or playing. The benefits of following a good warm-up routine – based around the exercises outlined on pages 22–33 – are twofold:
1. You will increase your performance at the start of a game or practice session
2. You will decrease your risk of injury.
There is also a psychological benefit to be gained from a thorough warm-up. If you feel that you are properly prepared, you will be confident and raring to go at the start of a game. Time spent warming-up can also help you focus on what lies ahead – composure is a valuable commodity at the start of a football match. Warming-up can also help to relax tense and nervous players.

A 15-minute warm-up will ensure you're properly prepared for the physical exertions which lie ahead, but if you fail to warm-up for long enough the results can be disastrous. Even if you are fortunate enough to get through the game without picking up an injury, you will be unable to perform at your maximum level from the start of the game. For the first 10–15 minutes, you will effectively be warming-up.

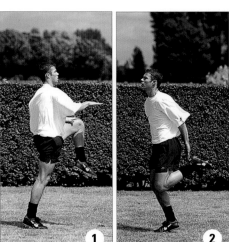 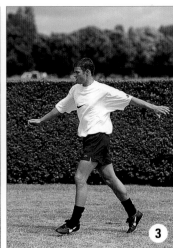

The three exercises shown above will get your heart-rate up and are a good framework around which to build your warm-up:
1. Kick your knees up high, using your hands as a guide.
2. Flick your heels up to touch your hands as you run.
3. Twist the top of your body and run side-steps, alternating to face both ways.

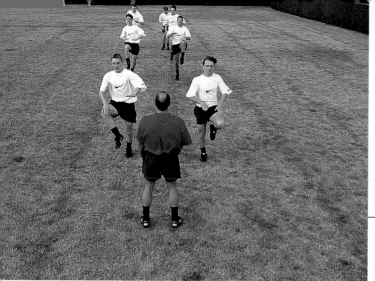
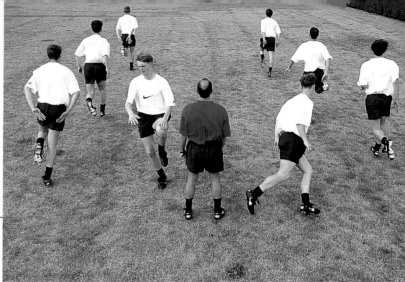

A WARM HEART

The warm-up also helps take your heart rate from a relaxed state up to a level at which it is ready for work. That level should be something in the region of 120 beats per minute. As the heart-rate goes up and the flow of blood around the body increases, your muscles produce heat. As the intensity of the warm-up is raised, more heat is generated and some is transferred from the muscles into the blood and dispersed throughout the body.

An organised team warm-up will ensure everyone is prepared for the start of the game and can fill the opposition with fear. Here the players run towards the coach kicking their knees up and then turn and run away from him, flicking their heels up as they go.

WASTED WARM-UPS

Once you have completed your pre-match warm-up, do not return to the dressing room and put your feet up before going back out for the kick-off. This will waste all the work you have just done – your heart-rate will drop and your muscles will grow colder and less flexible. Instead, you should keep your body warm – jogging on the spot or continued stretching will work. So keep the body moving, particularly during winter months when warm-up takes on a whole new importance.

ON THE BENCH

If you are on the substitutes bench, you should still warm-up as if you are starting the game. You never know when you will be needed. During the first half of the game, substitutes should jog and stretch every 10-12 minutes. Warm-up for 15 minutes straight after half-time and every 10 minutes after that until you are needed.

WINTER WARM-UPS

When the weather is hot, your body temperature and muscles respond quicker than during colder weather. During the winter months it is essential to warm-up with plenty of layers of clothes on. Only remove your layers when you are sufficiently warm. Don't try to warm-up in just your playing kit when it's freezing cold – you will not be able to get sufficiently warm. On very cold days, try to warm-up inside and only venture out onto the pitch when you have to.

Playing outdoor football in the winter always involves a risk of injury, so it is as well to train in a gym, doing weights or playing indoor five-a-side. Avoid going out in freezing cold temperatures if you can. But always be prepared to work yourself hard when training inside during these cold periods. Don't use the weather as an excuse not to train.

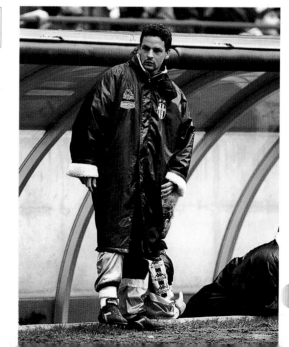

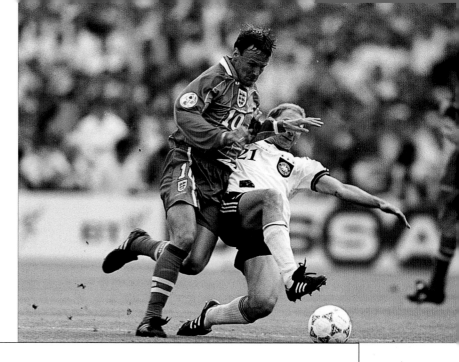

Professionals like Teddy Sheringham and Dieter Eilts have to train hard and prepare well to compete at the highest level. Here they tussle for a ball in the semi-final of the European Championships.

There isn't such a thing as a 'typical working week' for a professional footballer because training programmes vary according to circumstances. For example, a week when a team plays on Tuesday or Wednesday is different to a week with only a Saturday game. Fluctuation in the form of the team or the fitness of individual players can also dictate changes in practice and preparation. In order to simplify matters and give amateur players an insight into the world of professional football, outlined here is a seven-day programme suitable for a professional team with no midweek game. For reasons of time, this schedule could not be followed by an amateur team. However, the principles and methods employed should form the basis of any team's preparation. It is simply 'good practice'. A coach should try to blend elements of the professional programme into a schedule that is suitable for his team. And the closer he gets to the ideal week, the better prepared his team will be. A programme for a typical amateur team is recommended on pages 70—71.

a professional week

MONDAY

After a day off on Sunday, players should work hard on Monday afternoon. It is not a case of easing back into the working week. Having rested for 24–36 hours, and providing they have eaten the right things and looked after themselves, players' glycogen stores, which were used up on the Saturday, will have been sufficiently replaced during their rest period and they will be ready for a decent physical work-out. After a customary warm-up and stretch, the session begins with 20 minutes of low-intensity running. This is followed by ten minutes of high-intensity ball work and sprints, 20 minutes technical work with the ball and 20 minutes strength work. Training is completed with a warm-down session lasting seven to 10 minutes.

AC Milan (below) are one of the greatest club sides in the world. Their training and preparation is also second to none.

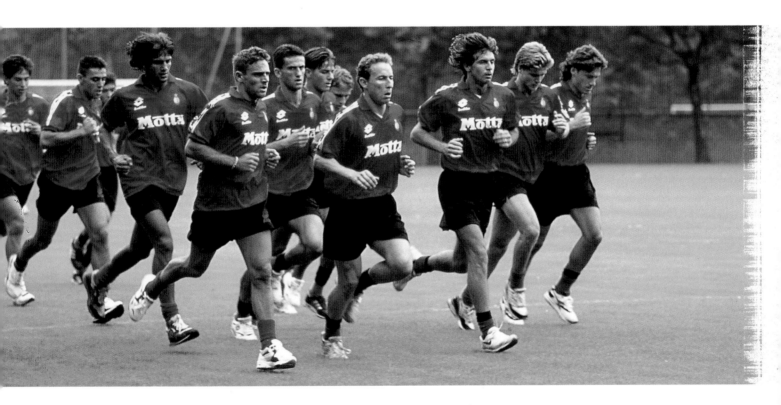

TUESDAY

A session of high-intensity work – before and after lunch this time. In the morning, after a warm-up and ten minutes of stretching, it's straight into 20 minutes of football-related rhythm running followed by 10 minutes of plymetric work. This is followed by 15 minutes of closing down routines – working the players hard in confined areas where they have to shadow their 'opponents'. The session is completed with five minutes of stretching off.

Following a light lunch and a brief recovery period, the afternoon session begins – again commencing with warm-up and stretches for ten minutes. Even though the players have warmed-up and trained in the morning it is still vital they go through the same preparation routine. After ten minutes of ball work in pairs, the squad divides into teams for two 20-minute games with the emphasis on tactics and technique. There are plenty of stops in these games as the manager halts play to get his views across. Afterwards, players warm-down.

With the correct training and preparation, part-time players have shown that they can compete with the top professional sides. Here Paul Warhurst of Blackburn Rovers is dispossessed in a midfield tussle with a Rosenborg part-timer during a Champions League clash in 1995.

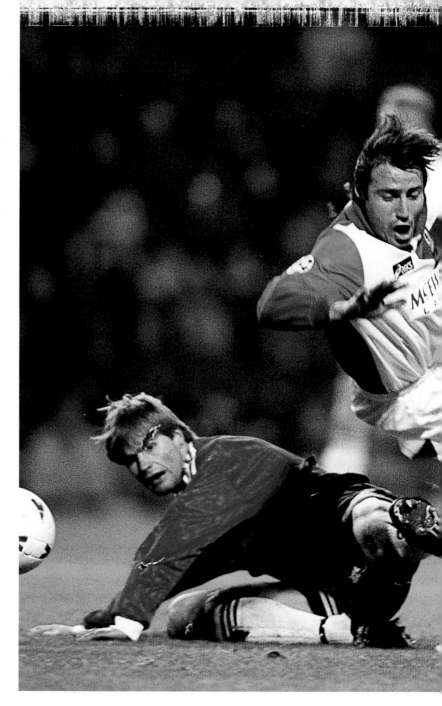

WEDNESDAY

At this stage of the week, a player's diet is crucial. He should be increasing his intake of complex carbohydrates, whilst taking on very little protein. There are no strict rules as to what a player should eat during the early part of the week, although obviously he should to eat sensibly. From Wednesday until Saturday, the recommendation is that he eats four small meals a day, supplemented with regular carbo drinks.

On the training front, players follow the following running routines:

1. 10 minutes slow running and stretching

2. 20-metre runs (six repeats with 30-second rest in between) building speed up gradually to 75% of maximum speed

3. 20-metre sprints (six repeats with 30-second rest in between) using various starts, including standard, backward and lateral running starts

This is followed by 15 minutes of plymetric work; a five-minute, high-intensity, small-sided game interspersed with five minutes of sprinting between cones before going back into a five-minute high-intensity game. The morning session is concluded with five minutes of high-intensity running followed by a 15-minute tactical game before breaking for lunch. After eating and resting, the players would return for 30 minutes of strength work in the gym.

THURSDAY

As matchday approaches, with the players having worked hard over the past two days, sessions are built around ball work.

But nothing is done without the customary ten-minute warm-up beforehand. A two-touch game of 35 minutes gives players a good work-out and allows them plenty of touches of the ball – very important at this stage of the week. Afterwards, 15 minutes is spent on crossing and finishing to give the strikers practice and sharpen up their touch in front of goal.

After lunch and a five-minute warm-up, there is a short session working on set-pieces – free-kicks, corners etc.

Remember, four small meals a day is much better for a player than two or three gut-busters. You do not want to undermine the good work you have done so far by eating the wrong things at the wrong time so close to match day.

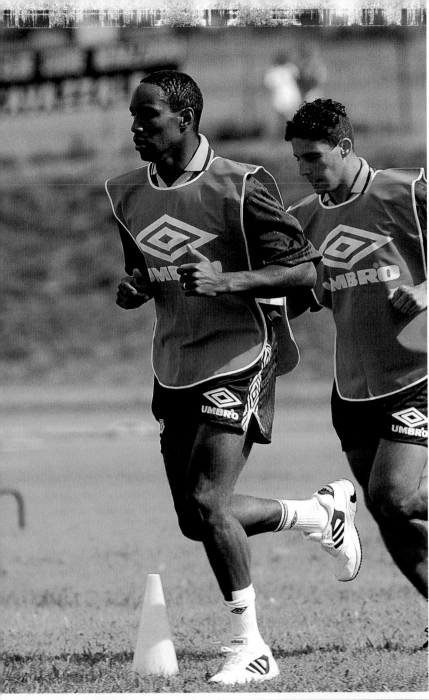

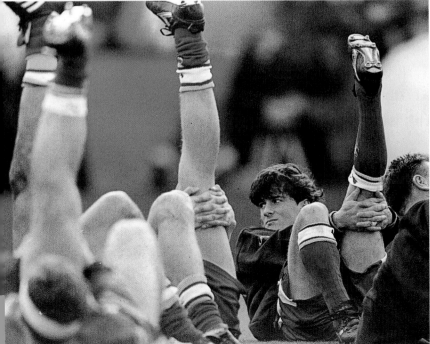

Left: Paul Ince goes through a gentle Inter Milan training session on the eve of a match. At this point training should not be too vigorous.

Bottom left: On matchday, good preparation is everything. Here Sheffield Wednesday limber up before a Premiership clash.

FRIDAY

With the match so close, a Friday training session should not be vigorous. The last thing a manager wants after a week of preparation is a player pulling up with an unecessary injury. After the usual warm-up, all the players should play a session of possession football – in a circle – for only 15–20 minutes. For the remainder of the day, players should pay special attention to their diet and concentrate on getting as much rest as possible for the next day's game. Any other form of strenuous exercise is out until 3pm tomorrow.

SATURDAY

Match day. Routines will vary depending on whether the match is at home or away. An away game will usually mean travelling on Friday evening and staying overnight in a hotel, whereas before a home game players are left to their own devices, reporting to the ground an hour or so before kick-off.

In preparation for the game, players should eat a breakfast of wheat cereal with skimmed milk or protein powder – both high in carbohydrates. Dried or fresh fruits are also recommended. Players should eat nothing during the four hours before kick-off – although fluids and carbohydrate drinks can, and should, be taken during this period.

At the ground, players start to follow their own pre-match routines; however all should go through a good warm-up session. Do not underestimate the importance of your preparation at this stage.

After 90 minutes of action, it all starts again. Ah, the life of a pro footballer!

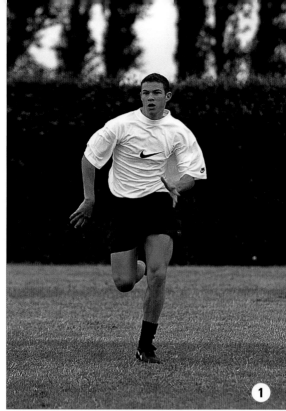

1

amateur week

Amateur players cannot attain the levels of fitness of professional footballers, but they can go close. In recent years part-time teams, particularly from Scandanavia, have upset many more illustrious, full-time professional teams in European competition. This goes to prove that, as an amateur, if you spend your time wisely and prepare properly it is possible to compete with the pros.

For most amateur players, a typical footballing week consists of two training sessions followed by a weekend game. While it is impossible to incorporate all the elements of a pro-week into this schedule, the principles remain the same and elements of the professional training programme can be employed.

FITNESS AND DIET

An amateur player can achieve a good level of fitness by training twice a week (for a maximum of two hours on each occasion), playing a game on a Saturday and following a few simple rules and tips along the way. For example, diet is just as important to amateur players as it is to the pros. In some respects it is even more important, as it is not easy for an amateur to compensate for dietary excesses with extra work on the training ground. The pressures of a nine-to-five job can also make healthy eating a low priority – all too often the amateur athlete is surrounded by unhealthy (though tempting) snack foods.

SOLO TRAINING

In addition to the training programme recommended below, amateur players should supplement their training with a weekly work-out in the gym to build muscle strength and improve anaerobic capacity. During spare time at home, simple exercises, such as sit-ups and stretches, can help keep the body supple and flexible.

TRAINING SESSIONS

The two team-training sessions should be divided equally between physical and technical elements.

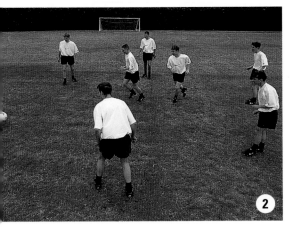

SESSION 1

The first session of the week – ideally on a Tuesday – should start with warming-up and stretching for at least 15 minutes. This is critical, as many players will not have exercised since the last game and muscles will take longer to loosen and warm-up in preparation of the exercise to come.

Follow the warm-up with four 300-metre runs around the pitch. This will raise the heart rate and improve aerobic fitness. This should be followed by two 15-minute games played at high intensity. These games will also help raise aerobic fitness. The intensity of games can be varied by switching between 'free football' and two-touch. Rest following the 15-minute games and then finish off the session with six 20-metre sprints followed by a warm-down.

A sprint exercise should also be on the agenda once a week. This will improve sharpness, acceleration and speed off the mark. Try and work the sprint exercise into the first training session of the week. This will leave more time in the second session to concentrate on the playing/technical side of the game.

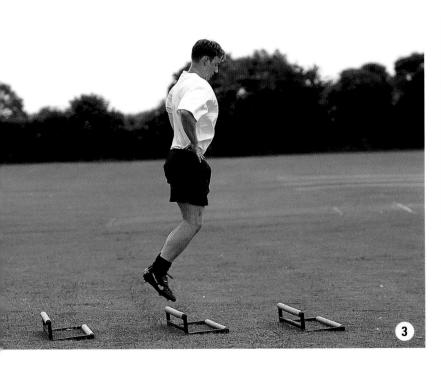

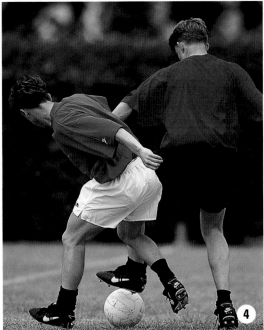

To make best use of the time your team has to train together, it is important to divide your sessions between physical and technical elements, as illustrated above:

Picture 1 – high-intensity running (see page 56)

Picture 2 – low-intensity ball-work (see page 63)

Picture 3 – plymetric training (see page 46)

Picture 4 – action from a high-intesity small-sided game (see page 56)

SESSION 2

In between the two training sessions, the amateur player should watch his diet and try some gentle running and stretching exercises to keep him in shape. The second session should be based around ball-work, improving technique and practice matches. But, of course, not without 10 minutes of warming-up before and warming down afterwards.

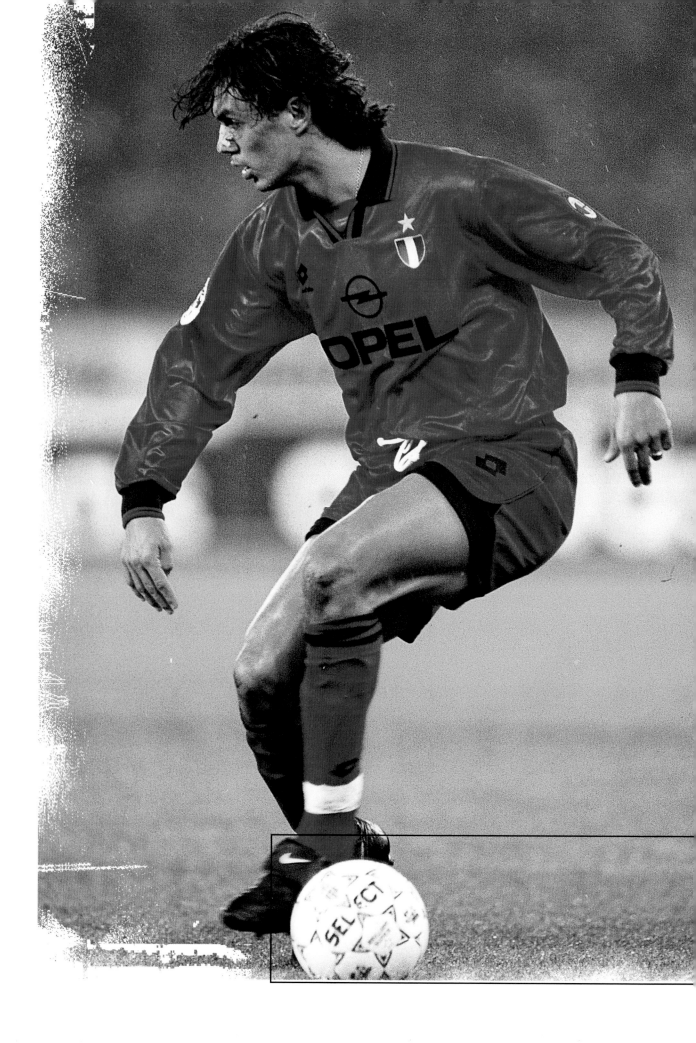

2
developing
your
technique

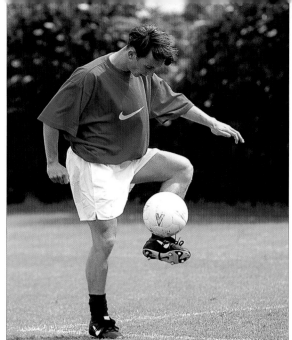

the skill factor

So far, we have concentrated on diet, preparation and fitness, however these things alone will not make you a top footballer. Ability, attitude and application all come into the equation. The key, however, is technique — without it a player's armoury is incomplete. You can be the fittest player in the world but, if you can't control and govern the ball, your fitness is worthless.

CONTROL AND PASS

Basic technique hinges on the ability to master a pass quickly and cleanly and deliver an accurate pass to a team-mate. 'Control and pass' is a phrase you will hear time and time again on training fields and unless you've mastered the art of control you cannot participate constructively in a game. Without the ball under your command and at your feet, moves will break down and possession will be lost. This is where fitness comes in, because you will have to work twice as hard to win the ball back. Not an ideal situation. Your energies are better concentrated on the basic arts when your team is in possession.

A lot of young players have the ability to keep the ball in the air (keepy up) many times but this is not the essence of control, although practising alone with the ball does help develop confidence and familiarity. 'Trapping the ball' is the platform from which to develop your technique and, as with everything we deal with in this section of the book, practice is essential unless you are one of those few people blessed with supernatural ability.

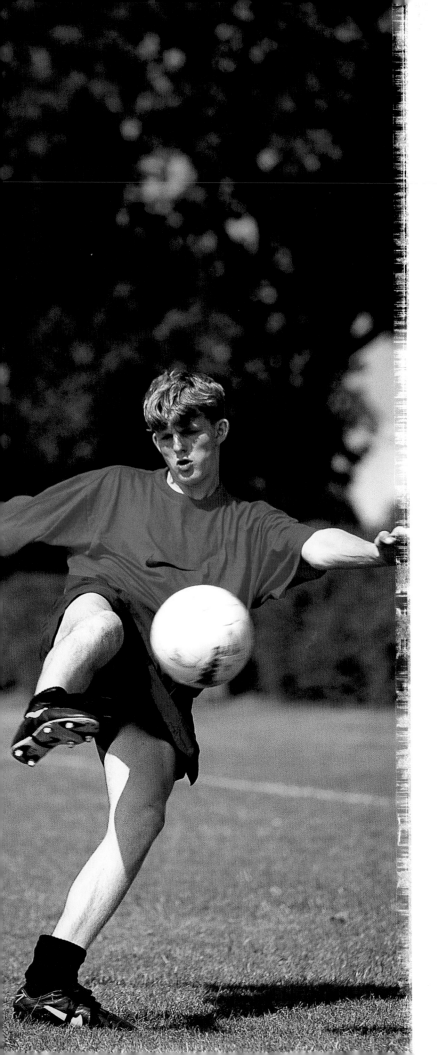

The only way to improve your technique is through practice. Skills like volleying are not instinctive, so if you don't work at them, you won't get any better.

YOUR GAME

You will hear coaches talking about your 'first touch' and, aside from the ability to actually strike a ball correctly and pass with pace and precision, this is so important. You can help develop this part of your game by turning to page 78. But control is not just about trapping or killing the ball with your feet. Other parts of the body are often called into play, such as the chest, head or even the thigh. The ball is not always going to be delivered to your feet, so you have to be prepared to try and bring if under control with other parts of your body.

In this section we also touch on aspects of the game such as dribbling, volleying, crossing and finishing. It is unlikely that you will master all of these arts, but it is important to have as many strings to your bow as possible. Advice on tackling, closing down and set pieces (free kicks, corners etc) complete the section and should provide a view of what goes to make a complete footballer.

With the modern game becoming more and more physical and fast, never has the need for a player to have good all-round ability and acceptable technique been greater. Read and learn and you could be on the way to becoming a better player.

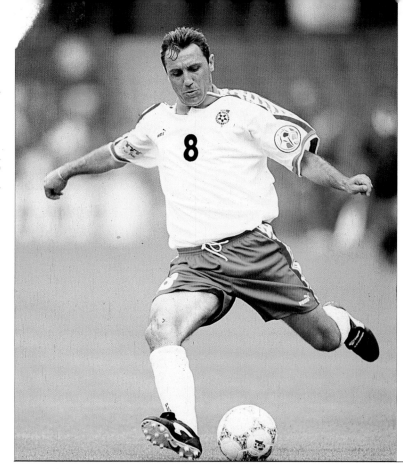

Hristo Stoichkov shapes up to hit one of his trademark left-footed drives. To make a good contact with the ball, you must get your body into a good position as you approach it.

If you can't kick a ball correctly, you're not going to go too far as a footballer. You may think this is obvious but, for many people, the most simple and basic aspect of the game does not come naturally. For some players it needs a lot of practice.

The more you play football, the more you realise the importance of keeping possession — the art of passing the ball to a team-mate with good weight and accuracy. To achieve that you need to feel comfortable with the ball at your feet and know when and how to deliver the ball to a colleague. This can only come when a player has developed the correct techniques and an understanding of where and when to apply them.

striking the ball correctly

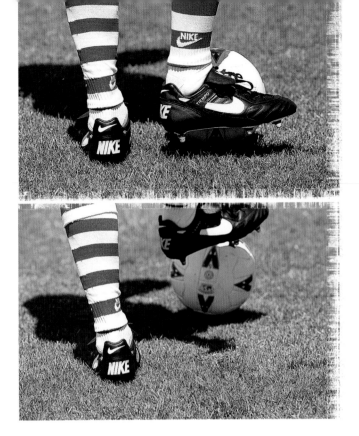

WHEN KICKING A BALL...

1. Avoid using your toe unless you have no other alternative.
2. When possible, try to use the inside, outside, top or instep of the boot (see below).
3. For the greatest degree of accuracy when passing – or controlling – the ball use the inside of the foot.
4. It is important to practise using both feet and not be dependent on one strong foot.
5. Position of your non-kicking foot correctly. It should always be next to the ball as it is struck and not ahead of or behind the ball. The position of your non-kicking foot determines the balance and power you generate.
6. Practise regularly and try to master the different ways – inside, outside or instep – of striking the ball. Using both feet too.
7. Check where you are aiming the ball before striking but remember to keep your eye on the ball when making the kick.

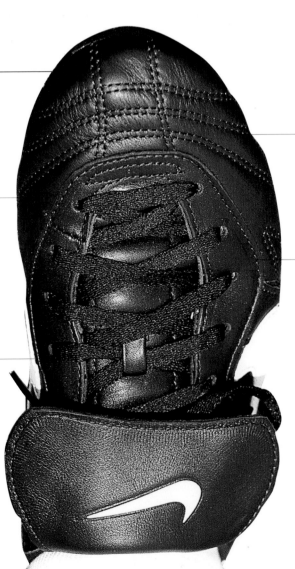

THE INSIDE
Probably the first area of the foot you will use for kicking. Used for controlling and passing the ball with the greatest degree of accuracy.

THE INSTEP
Used more often than any other part of the foot. Passing, crossing, chipping, shooting; the instep is used in the execution of all these arts.

THE TOP
The most powerful contact area of the boot. The sweet spot, as some like to call it. Used for driving the ball long distances, shooting or clearing.

THE OUTSIDE
Used for bending or swerving the ball around opponents, normally from dead-ball situations.

KICKING AREAS OF THE FOOT

Gica Popescu gets in position to control a bouncing pass. The art is to watch the ball onto your foot and to cushion it into your stride. If you master this skill, you will give yourself a yard on your opponents.

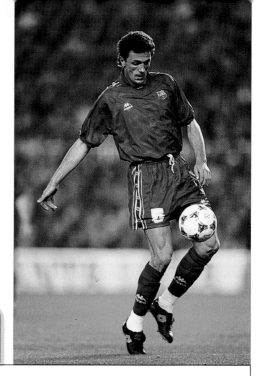

first touch

First touch is vital — watch any good player and you will instantly see the benefits of good control. The ball is under his complete control in an instant and, as a result, he has time to consider his next move. The pace of the modern game is such that you often only have a matter of seconds to receive, control and pass the ball to a team-mate. So don't waste time chasing a badly controlled ball. By developing a good first touch, you can give yourself time (even a fraction of a second could be important) to make an accurate pass and keep possession for your team. A bad first touch often results in the ball bouncing too far away from your body towards an opponent. Possession is almost certainly going to be lost.

The trap is one of the most effective, though dangerous, ways to control a ball. Effective, because if performed correctly the ball is under your complete control. Dangerous because if you lose concentration for a second, the ball will squirt away from underneath your foot. The key is to keep your eye on the ball.

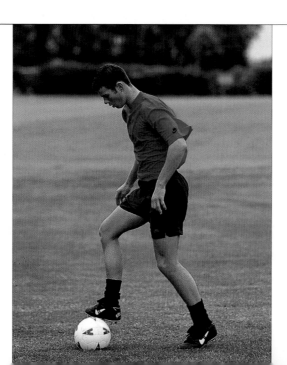

THE TRAP

Ball control is a basic art, yet one of the most effective when carried out correctly. The 'trap' is a fundamental method of controlling a bouncing ball and involves the use of the sole of the boot. It is a simple matter of raising your controlling foot high and bringing it down on top of the ball, killing the bounce and leaving you in possession. As always, keep your eyes firmly on the ball and try not to 'stamp' too firmly on it. Treat the ball as your friend, as many managers tell their players.

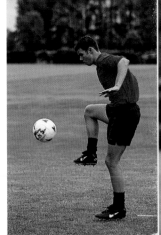

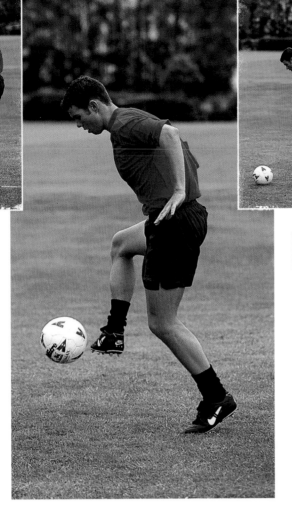

Controlling the ball using the inside of the foot is a fundamental skill. Watch the ball onto the large area on the inside of your foot, cushion it so that it drops into your stride and move away with it under your complete control.

SIDE OF THE FOOT

Another simple yet effective way of controlling the ball is using the inside of the foot – the side volley trap. Carried out correctly, this will cushion the ball and bring it to rest close enough to your body for you to make your next move. Again the key to this technique is keeping your eye on the ball, closely watching and judging its bounce and pace. Getting into a good, balanced body position before you receive the ball is also of paramount importance.

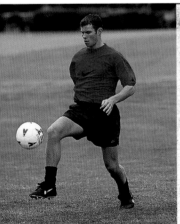

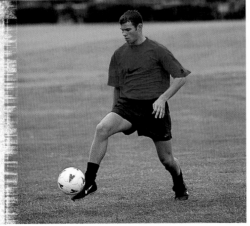

Using the top of the foot to control a high ball is a difficult skill. Keep your eye on the ball and pull it down as it hits your foot.

TOP OF THE FOOT

Using the top of the boot to cushion a high ball as it drops is another common practice, although marginally more difficult than the trap or side volley trap.

PRACTICE

SOLO PRACTICE
As with any aspect of the game, practice makes perfect and there are two simple ways you can improve your first touch. If you are practising alone, find a wall to work on your receiving techniques – striking the ball at various heights, speeds and angles to test your control. Many professional players will tell you how they practised like this for hours.

TWO-PLAYER PRACTICE
If you have a partner you can practise by kicking or throwing the ball to each other, from all distances, and work on the different ways of bringing the ball under control. Remember, your game will suffer if you have a poor first touch.

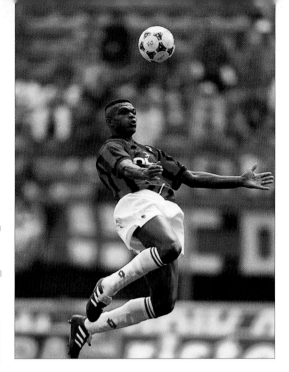

Frenchman Marcel Desailly controls the ball with a cushioned header. To bring the ball down in this way, you must lean back (to take the pace off of the ball) and direct the header downwards.

head, chest and thigh

In addition to using your feet, there are three other parts of the body which can be used to control a moving ball. The head, chest and thigh can be used to cushion the ball and take the weight out of a high pass. You are not always going to receive a pass along the ground, so it is important to know how to deal with a high ball and bring it to rest before an opponent has time to close you down.

CHEST AND THIGH

The technique for controlling the ball either on the chest or the thigh is much the same. It is all about watching the ball and cushioning it so that it drops nicely to your feet. When using the chest it is important to be in a good body position, on your toes and leaning back slightly as the ball makes contact with you. When the ball hits your chest it will begin to drop and you will be in position to complete the control with your feet.

When controlling the ball with the thigh remember to watch the ball until contact is made. Your thigh should be positioned at an angle of 45 degrees to the ground. Once again, cushion the ball and, as you bring your leg down, the ball will drop to your feet.

Whether you are planning to use your head, chest or thigh the most important things to remember are these:

1. Keep your eyes firmly on the ball (not your opponent) as it approaches you, watching it onto the part of the body you have chosen to control it.
2. Concentrate on getting your body into a good position to receive the ball. Balance is important, so make sure you are relaxed and not leaning too far forward
3. Make up your mind early and execute your move swiftly. Making the right decision and displaying good control will often enable you to avoid being tackled.
4. Practise.

It all sounds very simple and the truth is that football is a simple game.

HEAD

Using your head to control a high ball is more difficult. Being relaxed and well balanced is essential in this case. The aim is to cushion the ball with the front part of your forehead. Remember, you are not looking to head the ball any great distance so, as with the chest control, you should be leaning back slightly, watching the ball onto your forehead and guiding it back to the ground. You will then need to adjust your body position quickly to enable you to control the ball with your feet before moving on.

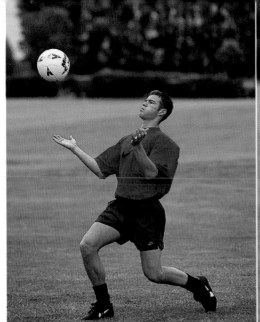

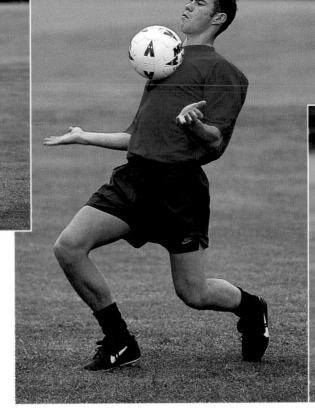

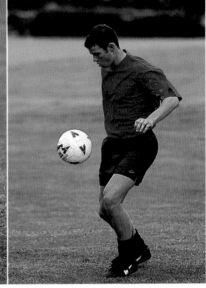

To control the ball on your chest, you must get into position as early as you can and watch the ball onto the large area of your chest. Lean back and direct the ball into your stride.

Thigh control is rarely used but it is a technique worth mastering. The key is to cushion the ball and pull it downwards, rather than push it up and away from your body.

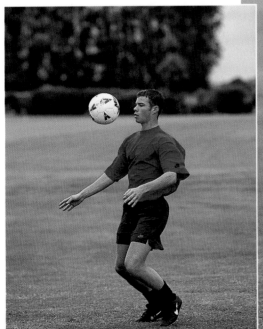

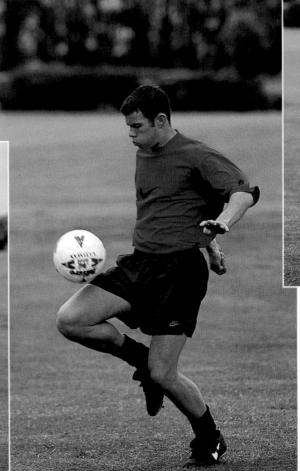

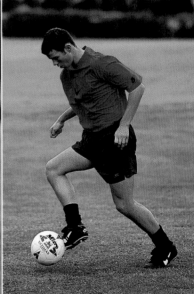

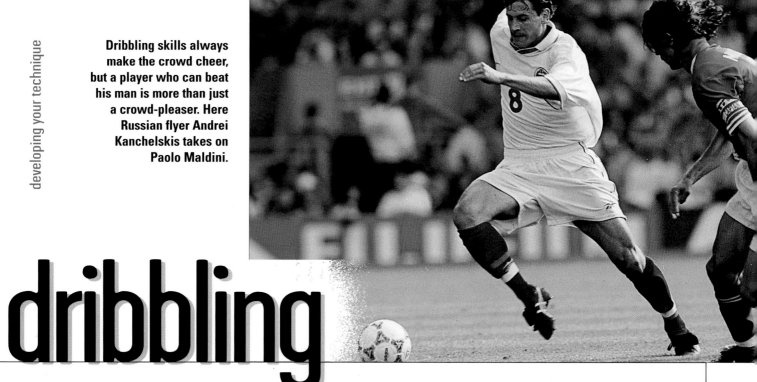

Dribbling skills always make the crowd cheer, but a player who can beat his man is more than just a crowd-pleaser. Here Russian flyer Andrei Kanchelskis takes on Paolo Maldini.

dribbling

Football is a team game but there is still plenty of room for individual skill to flourish. Let's face it, one of the great sights in football is seeing a skilful player go on a mazy, jinking run taking on and beating defender after defender. Dribbling with the ball, at speed, is a wonderful art — some would say a dying one in the modern game where so much emphasis is placed on team play. Nevertheless, dribbling is a potentially lethal part of a player's armoury....the ability to beat an opponent in a one v one situation.

A TIME TO DRIBBLE AND A TIME TO PASS

When you receive the ball you must usually decide what you are going to do very quickly. Pass to a team-mate or take on an opponent. There is no time for indecision or the moment will be lost.

The important thing is knowing when and in which areas of the field to take up the dribbling option. Don't, for example, try and beat two or three opponents on the edge of your own penalty area – not unless you fancy a dressing-down from a stressed-out coach. The final third of the field is the best area to chance your arm and turn on the style with a mazy dribble.

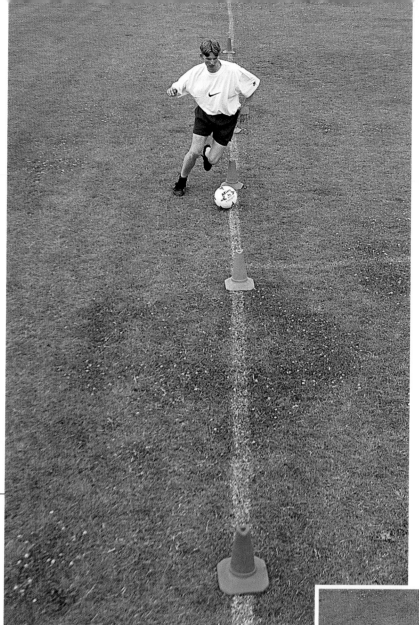

PRACTICE

Dribbling is very much an individual skill, so it's difficult to teach. But, by practising with a ball and a few cones you can develop your control and your own dribbling style. When practising, bear in mind a few key principles:

1. Make sure you have the ball under control before you begin your run, and keep it there during your attack.

2. Keep the ball close to your feet. Good dribblers seem to have the ball tied to their feet, making it very difficult for opponents to win it.

3. Keep your eye on the ball…

4. …but it is also important to keep looking up and continually weigh up your options.

5. Be confident.

Dribbling through cones is one of the best ways to perfect your skills. Concentrate on turning with the ball – to be truly effective, you must be able to turn both ways, otherwise you will become predictable.

TRICKS OF THE TRADE

One-v-one situations can be cat and mouse affairs, especially in the classic confrontations between wingers and full-backs. All the great dribblers have a vast repertoire of skills and tricks which they use to bewitch opponents. The step-over, the drag back, the scissors and many other exciting moves are the standard fare of top wingers. All of these skills should only be used once you have mastered the most effective and widely used dribbling technique: the body swerve. This move is simple in theory – you merely feint to go one way and then check back and take the ball in the opposite direction – but it takes a great deal of practice to perfect. The key to the body swerve is making the defender 'buy' the feint.

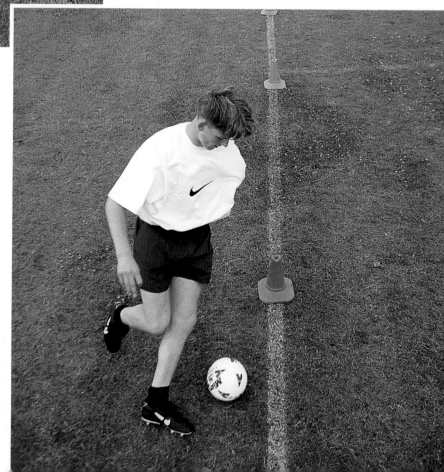

Skilful players like David Beckham
are able to hit bending, 50-yard
passes but still appreciate the
value of a short, side-footed pass.

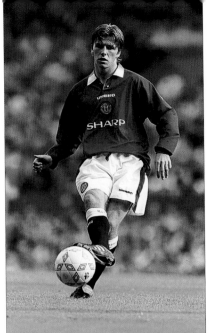

Skilful players like David Beckham
are able to hit bending, 50-yard
passes but still appreciate the
value of a short, side-footed pass.

side-foot
passing

Goals win games, solo runs excite fans, but the lifeblood of a football team is the art of good passing. In a nutshell, good passing is knowing where and when to hit the ball, with the right weight and accuracy. The quality of a pass is not measured by the way it is struck, but by the ease with which a team-mate is able to receive and control it.

There are many types of pass, not all of which you will be able to master, but the most important is the side-foot or push pass. This is the most reliable way of shifting the ball from one player to another. The kicking foot is turned out at right angles to the direction of the pass to secure a good contact with the largest available area of the foot. This pass is invariably used over short distances and it should be extremely accurate.

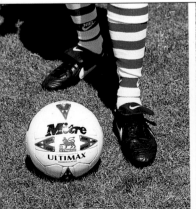
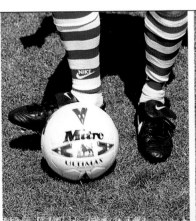
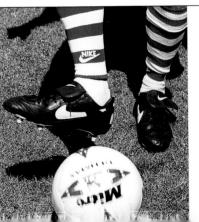

Side-foot passing uses the largest area of the side of the foot. Position your non-kicking foot next to the ball and strike through the ball. The follow-through will help dictate the weight of the pass.

Take time to practise your passing. Kicking a ball against a wall will help you to develop not only your passing, but also your control.

A passing circle (below, right) is another excellent way to hone your skills. Accuracy is everything, if your pass is badly directed or poorly weighted it will fail to make its intended target.

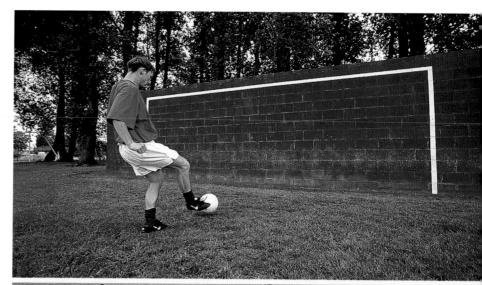

PASS MASTERS

The greatest passers in football, men like Glenn Hoddle, Ruud Gullit and Lothar Matthäus, have been as happy to use a short side-foot pass as a glorious 50-yard, high, bending pass. The side-foot is the most effective way of making sure your pass arrives at a team-mate's feet. There are three elements to a good pass: accuracy, weighting and timing.

ACCURACY is the most important aspect of passing because, without it, a move breaks down and your team loses possession. Your team-mates – and your coach – will appreciate you more if you can deliver the ball accurately. Don't try anything too ambitious, just make sure you retain possession – pass to a team-mate not an opponent.

WEIGHTING, i.e. the strength or speed of a pass, is critical. It's no good hitting an accurate ball to a colleague if there's too much pace on the pass. It will be difficult to control and is likely to result in possession being lost. Similarly, if the pass is too weak, the likelihood is it will not reach its intended target and will be intercepted.

TIMING, the art of knowing when to release the ball, is all down to good judgement and something only experience and practice can perfect.

If you combine these three elements with vision and perception, you will be an asset to any team.

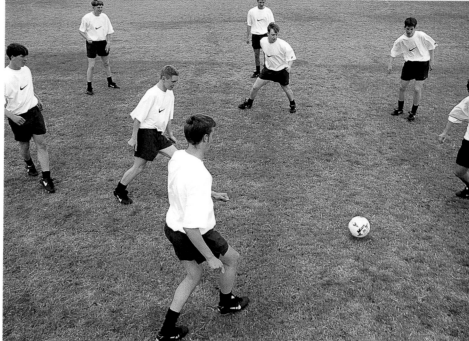

TIPS

- Stand upright and relax as you strike the ball
- If you are trying to hit a pass along the ground, do not lean back
- Use the large area on the inside of the foot
- Concentrate on the pace of the pass – a sloppy ball will play a team-mate into trouble
- Try to keep your body between the defender and the ball
- Don't switch off once you've made your pass. Run into position for a return ball. Pass and move, don't just stand and admire what you've done

advanced. passing

Side-foot passing is the safest and most accurate way of finding a team-mate. But it is not always an option open to you. If, for example, an opponent is standing between you and your intended target, a side-foot pass is likely to be intercepted. This is where the chip or bend pass come into play.

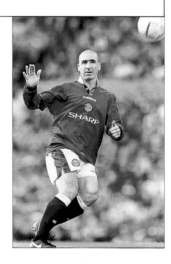

Eric Cantona delivers a delicately chipped pass. Skills like these take a great deal of practice.

THE CHIP PASS

The chip pass is more ambitious and the margin for error is greater, but there are times when it is very effective. It requires a fair degree of confidence. It can be used to put a team-mate into an attacking position, taking out an opponent in the process. It can also be used in a defensive situation when you are under pressure from a player closing you down. Either way, there are benefits although your technique needs to be spot on.

The correct way to play a chip is to make a 'stab' at the ball and get your foot right underneath it. Contact is made with the lower part of the instep and this has the effect of putting backspin on the ball and lofting it into the air. The chip needs just a short backlift of the kicking leg and hardly any follow-through. The key is to get enough height on the ball to clear your opponent while at the same time directing your pass accurately enough to find a team-mate. An early rise and a fast stop are two things you to look for in a chipped pass.

BENDING THE BALL

Bending the ball around an opponent – or a defensive wall at free-kicks – requires an entirely different approach, although the basics such as eye on the ball, good body position and balance still apply. The two major differences are that the side of the kicking foot makes contact with the side of the ball and, vitally, the follow-through is long. If you perform this skill correctly then the ball spins as it goes through the air and curves towards the player who is due to receive the ball. You must make sure to exaggerate the follow-through with the kicking leg. Without this follow-through you won't create enough spin to bend the ball around the opponent or wall.

The Brazilians, in particular, are past masters when it comes to the art of bending the ball. Great players such as Garrincha, Rivelino, Pele and more recently Zico and Juninho have baffled opponents – notably goalkeepers – with their ability to curve the ball with their infamous 'banana' shots.

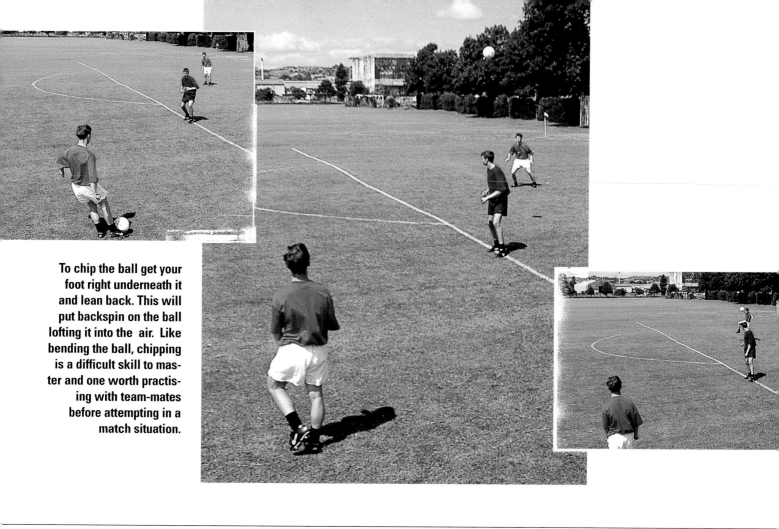

To chip the ball get your foot right underneath it and lean back. This will put backspin on the ball lofting it into the air. Like bending the ball, chipping is a difficult skill to master and one worth practising with team-mates before attempting in a match situation.

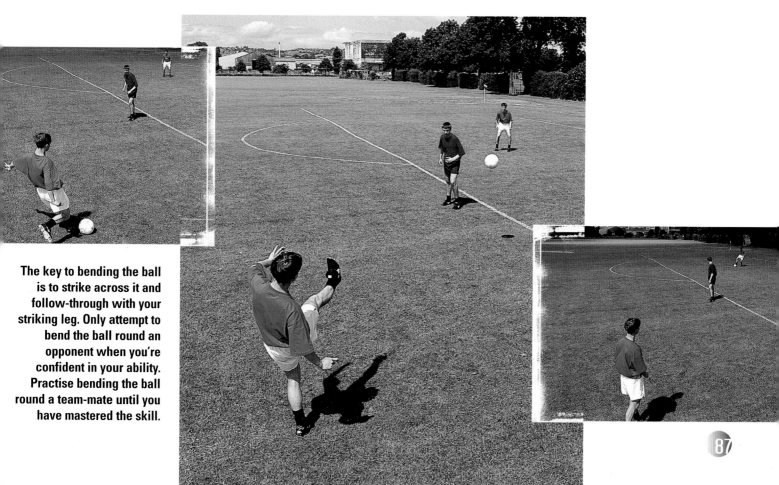

The key to bending the ball is to strike across it and follow-through with your striking leg. Only attempt to bend the ball round an opponent when you're confident in your ability. Practise bending the ball round a team-mate until you have mastered the skill.

Volleying is a precise skill. It is used when time and space is limited, usually as a hair-trigger reaction to a high pass or to take a snap-shot at goal. Striking the ball first-time, without the opportunity to control it, is a difficult technique to master and therefore requires a great deal of practice. There are many types of volley, but whether a player is attempting a low volley, high volley, half-volley, spectacular overhead or scissors kick, there is no margin for error. When it goes right, there's nothing quite like the thrill of striking a stunning volley into the back of the net. But when it goes awry, the results are ugly! As with most things, there is a time and a place for the volley, so pick and choose your moments to bring it into play.

volleying

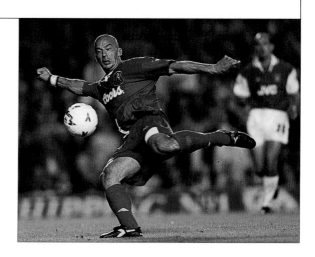

Italian striker Gianluca Vialli is renowned for his volleying technique. Here he lets fly in an English Premiership match.

PRACTISE LIKE THE PROS

The spectacular volley is the trademark of top players like Frenchman Eric Cantona and Italian superstar Gianluca Vialli. Both are genuinely gifted footballers who possess a high level of skill and an almost flawless technique. Yet they would be the first to admit that they still need to practise. Seeing Cantona on the training field when the rest of his team-mates have departed is commonplace. And, invariably, he spends a great deal of time perfecting the art of volleying. If players of the stature of Cantona and Vialli feel the need to practise the rest of us must work even harder. Practise hard and practise often if you wish to improve your volleying.

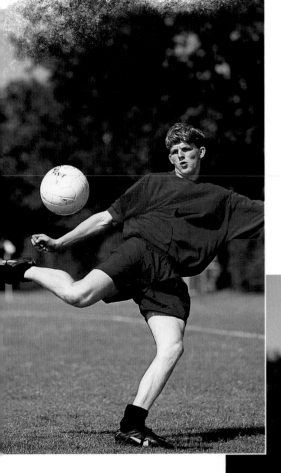

To keep your volleys down, you must get your leg above the ball, watch the ball onto your foot and follow-through. There is very little margin for error and when things do go wrong, the results can be embarrassing.

SHAPING-UP

When contemplating a volley one of the most important considerations, strange though it may seem, is the position of the non-striking foot. At the time of impact you are standing on one foot only and the power you can get into the shot will depend on how well you have positioned yourself.

To get maximum power in your shot you must bring the upper part of the striking foot into contact with the moving ball. Keep your eye firmly on the ball. Unlike bending the ball, the follow-through with a volley is not that long, although it is important to remember to keep the swing of your leg smooth and not to snatch at the ball.

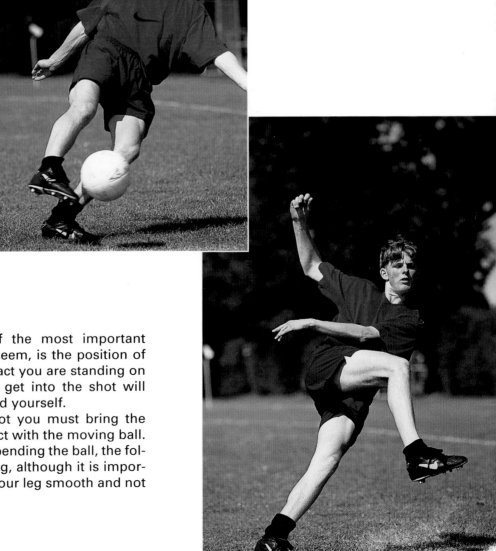

crossing

Football experts have suggested that up to 60% of goals come from crosses into the penalty area. According to a respected figure in modern football, 'the cross is one of the most important of all attacking techniques'. Whether you believe the numbers or not, the need to perfect this productive aspect of the game is obvious. For many years the art of crossing was restricted to wingers. Nowadays every outfield player must be able to make telling, intelligent crosses into the box. Overlapping full-backs, wing-backs and supporting midfield players must all be proficient when it comes to delivering varied and testing balls into the opponent's danger zone.

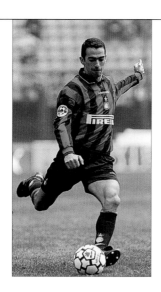

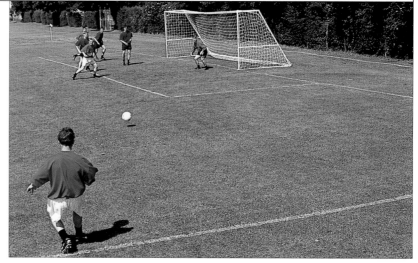

Left: Inter Milan's Djorkaeff drives in a cross. Accuracy is the key – don't just float over a hopeful ball.

Above: Vary your delivery; a low driven cross is often more dangerous than a high hanging ball.

HIT IT HARD

While you are practising – and even more so during games themselves – be positive and confident about the ball you are going to deliver. Crosses that float behind the goal or drop limply in the keeper's hands are frustrating for all concerned, particularly the striker who may have made a 50-yard run to meet your ball. Don't just dolly it into the box.

Ping your cross in with pace and purpose in equal measure.

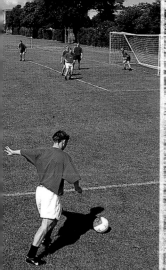

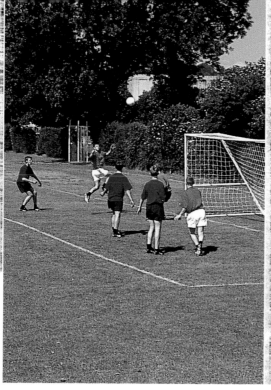

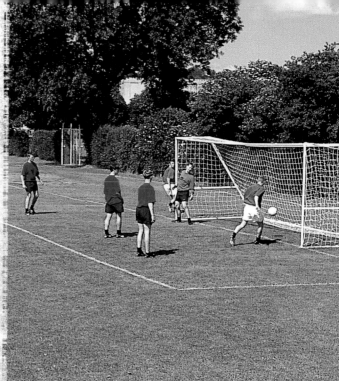

Most strikers thrive on balls delivered to the far post. But don't just float the pass over. Hit it with pace and give your team-mate something to get his head onto. It is also important to keep your cross away from the opposition goalkeeper.

STRIKING THE RIGHT BALANCE

Other critical factors to consider when crossing the ball are body position and balance. Delivering the ball on the run, in particular, is all about balance. When making the cross, spread your arms out wide to maintain balance and try to get your body facing the direction you're aiming the ball. Getting into this position is not always possible – sometimes you will be forced to cut the ball back from an acute angle. In this situation, keep your balance and composure. And keep your head down until contact has been made.

KEEP THEM GUESSING

Striking a football is very much like striking a golf ball. Lift your head before making contact and you are likely to top the ball and make a hash of the cross. Ask any good winger and he will also underline the importance of varying crosses – far post, near post, low, high, driven and looping. Do not become predictable by playing the same ball, however potentially dangerous, into the box time after time. Vary your delivery by knocking shorter balls into the near post rather than hitting everything long and high. Keep the defenders and the keeper guessing.

A MEASURED DELIVERY

There's more to crossing a ball than merely getting down the line and whacking it into the middle in the hope that your big centre-forward will get on the end of it. Before you send your cross over, you should consider the following:

1. Check you have at least one team-mate – hopefully more – in the box.

2. Choose your best option and try to pick that player out with an accurate ball.

3. The timing of your delivery is also important. Give a team-mate the best possible chance of making contact with your cross.

4. A driven cross is harder to defend against. A floated effort gives the keeper more time to come off his line and intercept.

5. The cross that is played in quickly from the bye-line causes more trouble than most.

6. Always try to swerve the ball – with pace remember – away from the keeper making it difficult for him to collect.

7. Keep your crosses away from defenders. There is nothing more frustrating than a cross that fails to clear the first defender.

8. The ideal place to aim your crosses is somewhere between the six-yard box and the penalty spot. Balls played into this area force keepers into a hard decision: do I come for the cross or stay on the line?

If you follow the above guidelines you will be well on your way to improving your crossing.

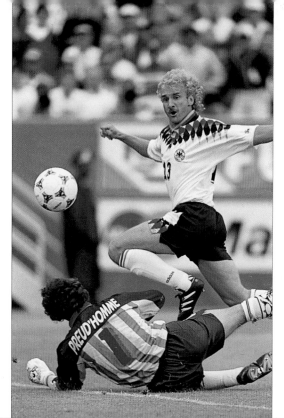

finishing

Scoring from close range is as much an art as crashing the ball into the top corner from 25 yards. In many cases it's a tougher prospect for a player to find space inside a crowded penalty area and still hit the target.

Above: German striker Rudi Völler keeps his cool to lift the ball over the advancing Belgian keeper Preud'homme during the 1994 World Cup finals.

Right: Lifting the ball over a keeper who has come off his line is one of the best finishing techniques for one-v-one situations. The key is to wait for the keeper to go down before you shoot.

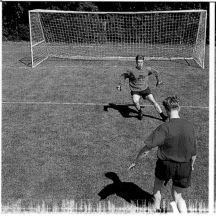
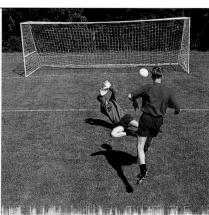

GET IN THE RIGHT POSITIONS

All strikers have some things in common, including a hunger and an eye for goal, and single-minded determination bordering on the selfish. Goalscoring inside the box, whatever the angle, requires speed of thought as well as movement. It calls for instant reactions – a split second can mean the difference between a blocked shot and a goal scored. Some players have an uncanny knack of getting into the right positions and finishing coolly. But all players, no matter how gifted, can increase their sharpness around the penalty area with practice.

Things happen very quickly in and around the 18-yard box, so players must work at developing an awareness of what is going on around them and react accordingly. Concentration is essential for strikers; they must be alert and on their toes at all times. A chance can go begging in a split-second. For this reason, strikers should spend plenty of time working on plymetric training, so that they can develop their reactions, and on anaerobic training to develop their acceleration.

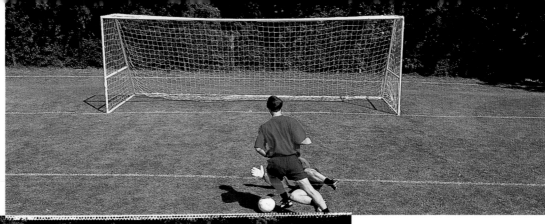

Dribbling around the keeper is a difficult skill. Try to keep your body between the ball and the keeper, thus making it hard for him to get to the ball without fouling you.

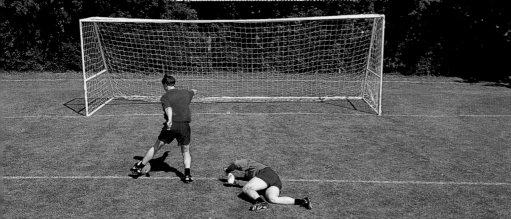

Take the ball around the keeper, once he is committed. But try not to get forced too wide – otherwise you might end up having to shoot from a tight angle.

Don't rush and don't 'showboat'. There are no speed bonuses and no extra points for artistic merit. Simply keep your shot down and into the middle of the goal – hit it firmly but don't blast it.

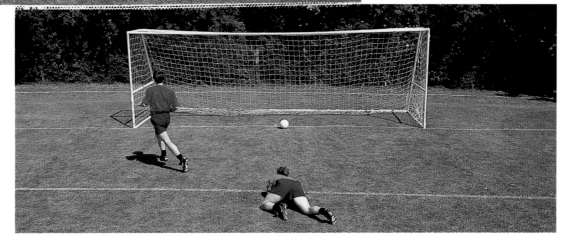

FINISH COOLLY

Once you've developed the fitness and awareness to get into goalscoring positions, you must take care not to squander your opportunities. Keep looking around you and take note of where your team-mates are – you may want to play a one-two, use a colleague as a decoy or get in a position to receive a pass. If the ball breaks to you, you must be instantly aware of your options and exploit them to the full. Try to find space, where possible, and know where the keeper is standing.

By correctly reading a situation, you may give yourself an extra yard over an opponent (plymetric and anaerobic train-ing will also help you react first). Once you are in possession of the ball you must remain composed – act quickly, but don't be hurried. Decide what you are going to do and don't change your mind. A moments hesitation will be costly. Decide where you are going to put the ball and strike it with confidence. And remember, you don't have to blast the ball to score. The legendary Jimmy Greaves scored hundreds of goals by 'passing the ball into the net'. He even struck his shots with a minimum amount of back lift to save a split second of time. You should try to vary your finishing – chip, drive, side-foot, outside of the foot. Consider your position, make your mind up and slot it in!

heading

Heading the old heavy footballs with their hard laces was a danger-ous business, but nowadays the modern ball poses no such threat. There is no good reason to avoid an aerial challenge...it's just a matter of confidence. Beat the fear and get your head on the ball.

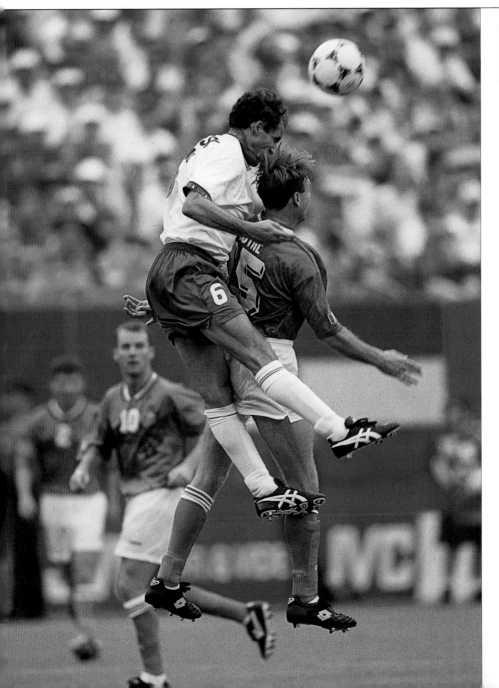

SHORT OR TALL, HEAD THE BALL

Heading is one of the most neglected skills in football. It is also an extremely valuable skill. A player who is strong in the air is an asset to any team, but a play-er who can't head a ball, no matter how good he is on the ground, will never make it to the top. Only in five-a-side is the ball played exclusively along the ground, during a typical 11-a-side game the ball will be airborne for 20% of the time it's in play. If you can't compete when the ball's not on the deck, you're a passenger to your team. But don't despair, anyone can learn to head the ball. It's a technique that requires practice and, at first, a little courage!

You don't have to be a giant centre-forward or centre-back to be a good header of the ball. Of course, there are times when being tall makes the difference between winning and losing an aerial challenge. But there's more to the art of heading than just being tall. Some shorter players are excellent headers of the ball. By the same token some tall players find it hard to win aerial challenges. Positioning and timing are just as important as standing height.

Heading is not just a skill for tall players. Aerial ability is as much about positioning and timing as standing height. Here, Franco Baresi shows excellent technique to beat a taller opponent.

THE ART OF HEADING

The skill of heading sounds simple enough, but is quite a complex art and many players, even top pros, fail to master it. The key to heading is making sure that the forehead is the point of contact. A common mistake is to use the top of the head. A mistake that many players, especially young ones, make is to close their eyes just before the moment of contact. Even some pros are guilty of this error. The proper way to head a ball is to get into position beneath the ball as early as possible, and to watch it onto your head. It is critical to keep your eyes open if you are going to make a good contact and give yourself the best possible chance of directing the header towards goal or a team-mate.

The neck muscles also come into play. Tense them as you bring your head back before 'attacking' the ball with power. Get the technique right and you will be surprised how much power and pace you can generate from a header. Also concentrate on judging the flight of the ball be aware of who is around you and use your whole body to elevate yourself.

CONFIDENCE

For all players, the most important thing to conquer is the fear of going up for a high ball. In the past there were real dangers in heading footballs. The ball was made of thick heavy leather and was held together by a lace. During the course of the game the ball would absorb water and become even heavier. Heading a ball like this could knock a man unconscious if he caught it wrong, and if the lace holes caught a player on the head he could be left with a nasty gash. Nowadays, footballs are coated with vinyl to protect them from the wet and have no lace holes, so the risks of getting injured by the ball when heading are minimal.

The best way to improve your heading confidence is to practise jumping and heading a suspended ball (place a ball in a carrier bag and suspend it on a rope). Once you are happy heading a ball unchallenged, you must develop your heading in practice games and matches. The important thing is to jump with purpose and be confident you are going to win the ball. Be strong and be decisive.

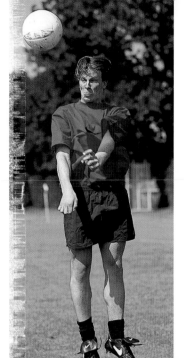

Keep your eyes on the ball – do <u>not</u> be tempted to shut them. Try to time your jump so that you are either above the ball if you want to head it down, or below the ball if you want to head it upwards.

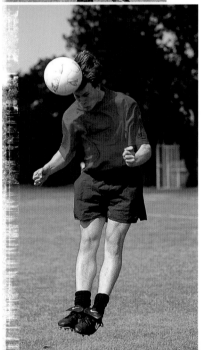

Strike the ball with your forehead and push it in the required direction. Try to keep your balance and brace yourself for the physical challenge of opponents.

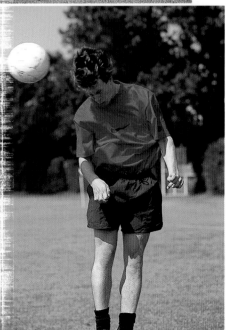

Use the power in your neck and upper body to get distance on the header. Follow-through once you have made contact with the ball.

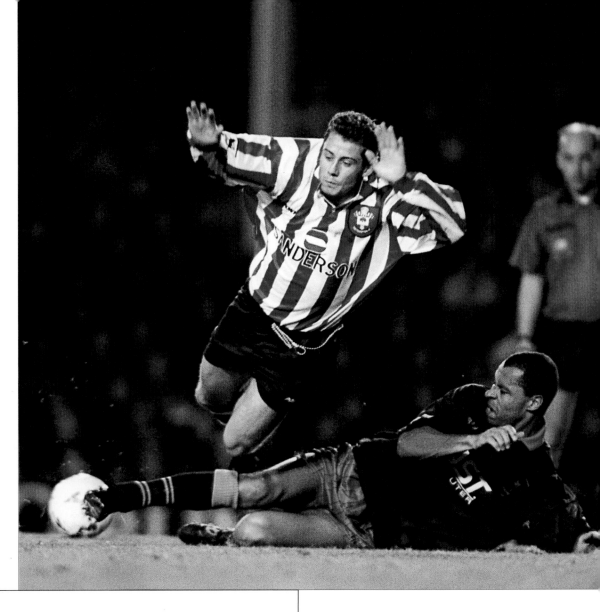

A split-second is the difference between a great tackle and an ugly foul. Here defender Paul McGrath demonstrates excellent timing to disposess an opponent.

If you don't have possession of the ball, you are not going to score...unless, that is, you are playing against very charitable opposition with a tendency to score own goals. When you lose possession, the whole team must work to cover, close down and, most importantly, win the ball back.

tackling

A SKILL FOR ALL

Many people take tackling for granted, but it is a real skill and needs to be practised. A good tackler will win the ball cleanly and will rarely give away a free-kick. A poor tackler will impatiently lunge in – often missing the ball or, more likely, catching both ball and opponent. Diving or sliding in is a waste of energy and can give away dangerous free-kicks and penalties or lead to injuries.

A well-timed tackle, like a goal, can be the difference between a victory and a defeat. A last-ditch tackle, made cleanly and clinically on the six-yard line, can avert a certain goal while a poor, ill-timed tackle can result in a penalty and a goal for the opposition. It is important, therefore, that every player in the team – even the goalkeeper – knows how to tackle. It is not just a defender's skill.

THE ART OF TACKLING

The art of tackling is to win the ball cleanly and either come away with it in your possession or put it out of play and out of danger. It has nothing to do with wild lunging challenges. Timing is central to good tackling; you must know when to make your attempt to win the ball. Don't commit yourself to the tackle too soon or you could be left on your backside with your defence exposed. Consider the position of your fellow defenders; committing yourself when you are the last man can be disastrous. Instead of lunging in, you should try and hold your opponent up and wait for team-mates to get back. In all cases, you should 'jockey' (hold up) your opponent until you feel the moment is right to pounce. Only make your tackle when you think you have a good chance of coming away with the ball. But when you have made up your mind to tackle, you should be decisive. Make a solid challenge and make it count. Half-hearted challenges not only give your opponent a better chance of keeping possession, but can also result in injury. Never just dive in.

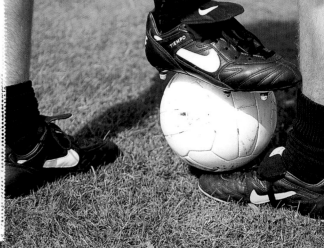

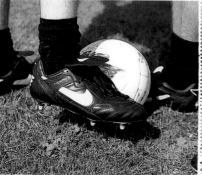

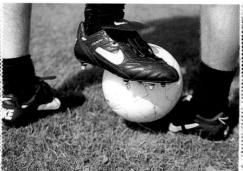

To win a block tackle you must get more of your foot on the ball than your opponent. Make a firm, but controlled, contact and push the ball over the top of your opponent's foot.

THE SLIDE TACKLE

The slide tackle is another option for winning the ball, but it requires perfect timing and if it goes wrong can be dangerous. It is not an option for the inexpert, as it frequently results in the opponent being brought down, and if the ball isn't won a free-kick is conceded – maybe even a booking if the tackle is from behind. However it can be devastating, particularly when executed by England's Peter Beardsley who makes a habit of winning balls in attacking areas of the pitch from surprised defenders. The key is to keep pace with the opponent and slide in when he least expects it, nicking the ball from him before you nick him and bring him down. You must make the tackle so that you can be on your feet and away with the ball before the opponent has a chance to recover himself. Beardsley seems to do it all in one fluent movement.

THE BLOCK TACKLE

The most common tackle in football is the 'block tackle'. This is when two opposing players arrive for the same ball at the same time. When you reach this 50-50 situation it is vital that you don't 'pull-out' of the challenge at the last minute. This can result in injury. Meet your opponent with a strong tackle, getting your body weight over the top of the ball to add to the strength of your challenge. Good body position and a bit of determination ensure that it doesn't always have to be the bigger, stronger player who emerges with the ball.

closing down

The aim of closing down is to give an opponent who has the ball as little time and space as possible to play it and find a team-mate. But, for closing down to be effective, you have to make sure that the whole team is covering and marking all of the opponents. If the man being closed down has one easy outlet, your hard work will be in vain.

WORK AS A TEAM

Whenever possession is lost the immediate priority is to win the ball back which means getting yourself into a position to make a tackle or block a pass. Closing down is the first stage on the way to winning the ball back. For it to be effective the whole team must work together and force an error out of the opposition – this can be a poor pass which is intercepted or poor control which gives the opportunity to tackle.

The man who has received, or is receiving, the ball must be put under pressure. He must be allowed no space or time to bring it under control and decide his options. The important thing is not to dive in. Try to hold your opponent up and, if you can, channel him to run with the ball on his weaker side; this may bring about a piece of poor control and a tackling opportunity.

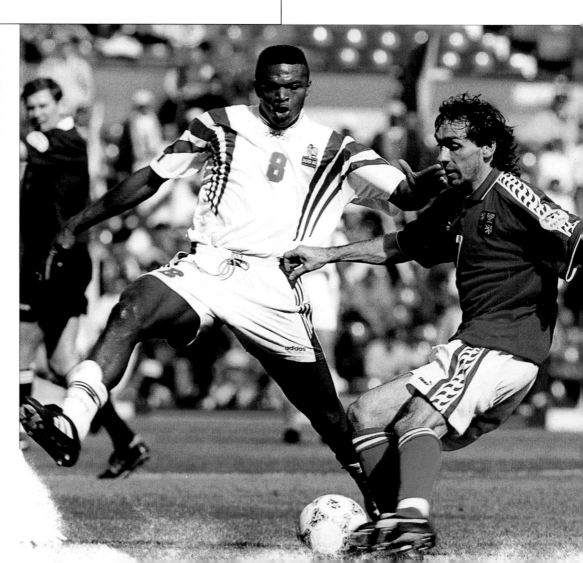

Frenchman Marcel Dessailly has closed down his opponent and forces him into a pass which will be easily blocked

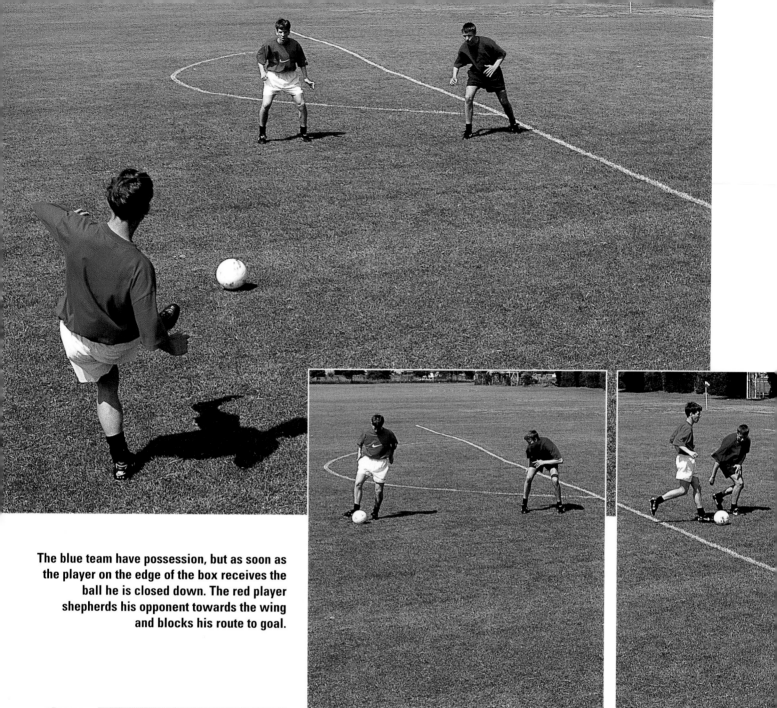

The blue team have possession, but as soon as the player on the edge of the box receives the ball he is closed down. The red player shepherds his opponent towards the wing and blocks his route to goal.

TIPS

- Be aware of all opponents, and not just the man in possession
- If you are not in a position to tackle, close down the space
- Stay on your feet and do not commit yourself to a challenge which you will be struggling to make
- Encourage team-mates, especially when they are looking tired
- Don't go so tight to an opponent that you make it easy for them to roll around you and turn you
- Defend from the front and defend as a team

A WORTHWHILE TASK

Closing down and tracking are tasks that appear unglamorous, but this type of hard work is highly valued by players, coaches and managers. All the best players work hard for their team and make efforts to win possession back when the ball is lost.

free-kicks

It is estimated that around a third of all goals are scored from free-kicks taken around the penalty area. Considering this statistic, it's little wonder that professional clubs practise these dead-ball situations on a regular basis in training. If you're skilful enough, a free-kick near the 18-yard box is a goal-scoring opportunity. Even with a solid and well-positioned wall and an agile goalkeeper these positions can lead to goals...you just need to know what you're doing.

Frank de Boer lines up to take a free-kick for Holland against Wales in a World Cup qualifier. Free-kicks from central positions like this are particularly dangerous as the keeper will not know whether to expect a shot into the left or right-hand corner of his goal.

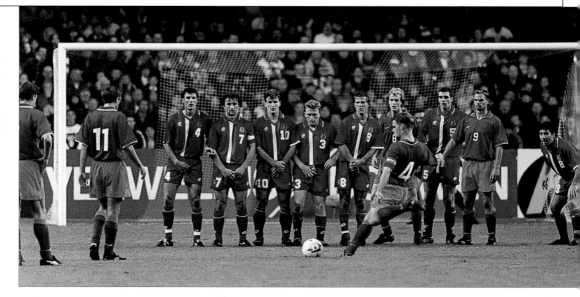

OPPORTUNITY KNOCKS

It may sound easy to score with an unchallenged shot from the edge of the box, but when there are 11 opponents – plus a few team-mates – between you and the goal the task is not so simple. In most cases, the defending goalkeeper will arrange a wall between him and the ball, before taking up a sensible position himself. Faced with a defensive wall 10 yards away, and a goalkeeper positioned so as to guard the unprotected area of the goal, a shot which is likely to beat the keeper has to be accurate and well struck. The most obvious way of scoring direct

from a free-kick is by bending the ball 'around' the defensive wall using the techniques outlined on page 86.

A ball hit with pace is more likely to beat a goalkeeper. But the distance from goal, the position of the wall and keeper may not allow you to do this. In these cases a chip, or a floated shot over the wall – aiming for the corner of the goal may be the answer. Either way, free-kicks require an endless amount of practice if they are to have a chance of coming off in matches. Even if you are not the team expert, you should still practise your free-kicks.

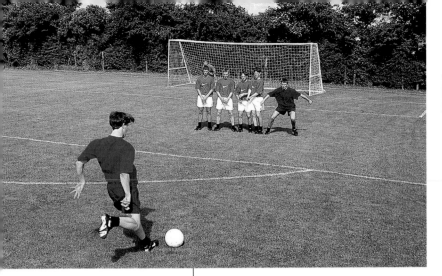

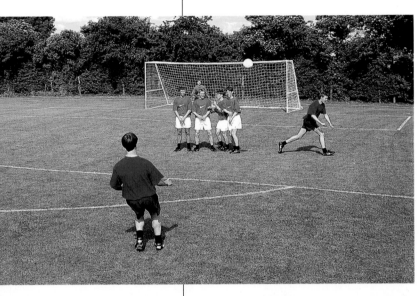

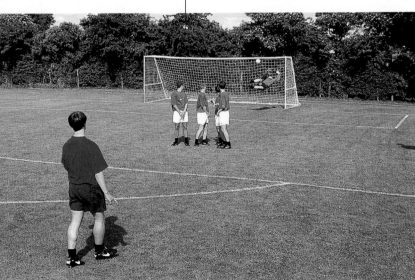

This popular free-kick routine is difficult to defend against if performed accurately. An attacker (in red) is positioned on the end of the wall and as the kicker approaches the ball, he peels off of the wall. The ball is then played over the gap left by the red decoy and into the corner of the net. Like all set pieces this routine must be practised before use in a match.

'BANANA KICK'

The South Americans are the past masters when it comes to curling free-kicks. As far back as the the 1950s Garrincha started the trend with his famous 'banana kick'. The theory is simple, you aim the ball wide of the goal, around the wall, but with enough bend to bring it back on target and into the net. In practice it is not that simple and like all football skills practice is exactly what you'll need if you want to perfect the 'banana kick'.

BASIC TECHNIQUE

• Assess the position of the wall and the keeper.
• Pick the spot where you intend to put the ball – and stick to it.
• You should be looking to place the ball just inside one of the posts, in other words as far from the keeper as possible
• In order to do this, aim the ball a couple of feet outside the post and allow the curl you put on it to bring the ball back.
• If you're right-footed, strike the ball with the outside of your foot to bend it from left to right and with the inside of the foot to bend it right to left.
• Strike the left half of the ball to bend it away to the right.
• Graze your foot across the ball and exaggerate the follow-through with your kicking leg.

DEVELOPING YOUR FREE-KICK

• Concentrate on accuracy first.
• Once you are consistently hitting the target, try to get the ball to bend.
• The final stage is to increase the pace of your kicks...but without losing accuracy.

free-kicks 2

Not all free-kicks (those for obstruction, for example) around the box are direct and some are from such an angle that a shot at goal is not a serious option. But any free-kick in the last third of the field, irrespective of the angle, is potentially dangerous.

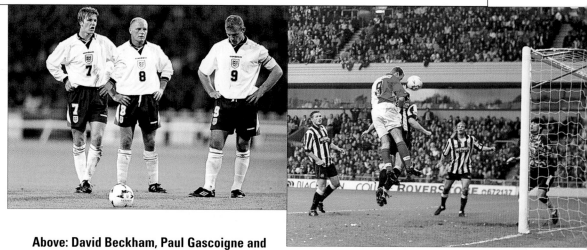

Above: David Beckham, Paul Gascoigne and Alan Shearer consider their options. Don't just hit a hopeful shot or an aimless cross. Take your time and consider your options.

Right: Great strikers like Alan Shearer (playing for Blackburn Rovers here) can make any ball into the box look good, but don't depend on your strikers to turn a poor free-kick into a goalscoring opportunity.

TAKE YOUR TIME

The worst free-kicks are those taken quickly by a player seeking to catch defenders out of position. In most cases, his team-mates are not ready either. The first rule of free-kick taking is 'think before you act.' Time is on your side, so go through what was rehearsed on the training ground. Nothing infuriates a coach more than a free-kick, practised and rehearsed over and again in training, but not employed in a match. Remember, it is the defending team which has the problem. Don't solve it for them.

KEEP IT SIMPLE

Do not try to over-complicate free-kicks. A complex move involving four players, one stepping over the ball, one touching the ball, another stopping it and finally the last player hitting it may look technically mind-blowing but will, more often than not, be ineffective. The more players involved the greater the chance of the move breaking down, preventing you getting a shot in on goal. You also give your opponents more time to close down. A simple touch to the side, to take the ball away from the wall, and a clinical shot from a team-mate is more likely to bring a positive result than an elaborate routine.

THE PASSING OPTION

If the defending side has put five or six men in the wall there is a good chance they will be outnumbered elsewhere in the box. There is a good chance of finding a team-mate in space in the area, so consider this option: a goal-scoring opportunity can result from an astutely taken short free-kick to an unmarked colleague.

Play to your strengths and don't waste the opportunity. If you have a neat skilful player, try to play him into the penalty area; he may be able to get a shot in, or, he may tempt an opponent into a wild tackle and earn you a penalty. Alternatively, if you have players who pose a threat in the air, put the ball in high. However, don't become too predictable; vary your delivery.

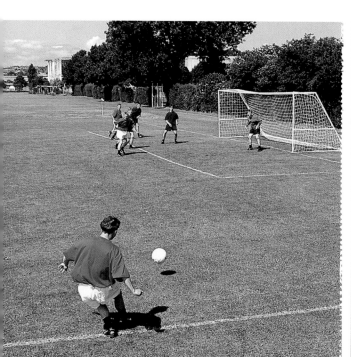

In this situation everybody expects a high-ball to the far post. However in this case the ball is delivered hard to the near post. The attacker catches the defenders napping and sneaks in to score.

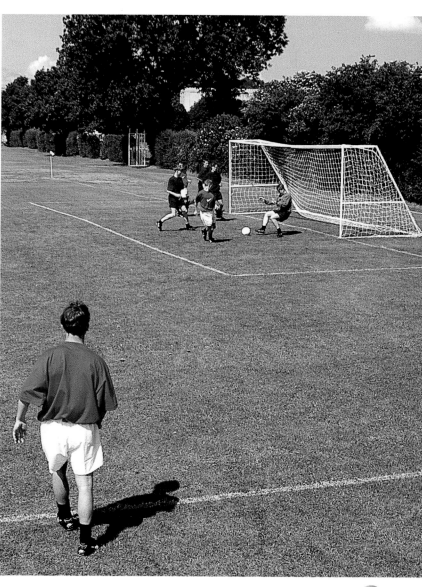

penalties

The best players do not necessarily take the best penalties. It is usually the player who holds his nerve best who is the penalty king. The basic skill of beating a goalkeeper from 12 yards is not difficult, but in the context of a highly competitive football match it can be daunting. And with the introduction of penalty shoot-outs to settle cup matches there are more and more of these nerve-tingling scenarios.

MAKE YOUR MIND UP

Decide where you are going to strike the ball before you put it down, and don't change your mind. Indecision is likely to result in a poor penalty. Only step up to strike the ball when you are composed enough to be confident that you will strike the ball well enough for it to reach it's intended target – the back of the net.

CONFIDENCE AND NERVE

A player can practise taking penalties all day long, but there is little to prepare him for being thrust into a position where victory or defeat is down, solely, to him. It can be a frightening prospect. Who would have liked to be a player in the shoot-out for the 1994 World Cup in the USA, or in the semi-final of Euro 96? The pressure must have been immense. Some players thrive on that 'winner takes all' situation, preferring to consider the prospect of scoring and being hailed a hero than missing and being damned as the villain. Confidence and a positive attitude; they are the two things which set penalty takers aside.

Alan Shearer holds his nerve to tuck away a penalty against Holland during the 1996 European Championships. At international level, the standard of goalkeeping is so high that there is little margin for error.

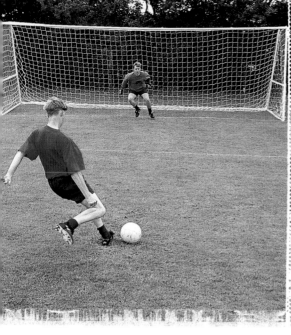

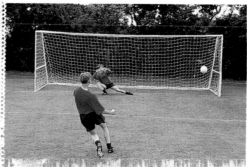

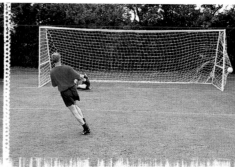

...in fact the ball is struck firmly into the opposite corner, giving the keeper no chance to make a save.

On the approach to this penalty, the taker has managed to deceive the keeper into thinking he is going to shoot to the keeper's right...

WHERE TO AIM

Whatever you do, try to keep your head down. There is nothing worse than skying a penalty over the bar. At least if you make the keeper save the ball there is the chance of a rebound. The closer you place the ball into the corners, the more difficult it will be for even the best goalkeeper to save it.

Most players favour the 'placed' penalty, struck low with the side of the foot into your chosen corner of the net. Some players, Republic of Ireland international John Aldridge for one, have perfected a little shimmy on the run up; this entices the keeper to commit himself before the ball is struck. There is an element of risk in this approach and it requires supreme confidence. Care must be taken not to break your run up though.

In recent years the 'blasted' penalty has become a popular option amongst certain strikers. The majority of keepers tend to commit themselves to a desperate, full length dive either way, so a direct route down the middle of the goal, using power, can be effective. If you choose this option, you must keep your head down and over the top of the ball to prevent your shot flying high over the crossbar.

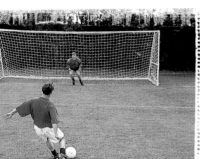

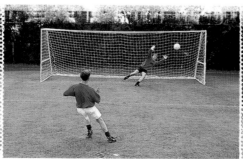

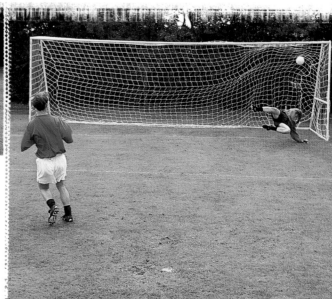

If the ball is struck accurately enough, it doesn't matter which way the keeper goes. Here the ball is hit into the top corner and even though the keeper goes the right way he has no chance.

throw-ins

Throw-ins are an important part of the modern game. In recent years, certain players have developed their throwing to such an extent that a throw-in anywhere in the opponent's half constitutes a goalscoring opportunity. The long throw is employed by many teams and can be as dangerous as a corner kick. Most full-backs will try to develop a long throw as it is such a tremendous asset to their team. Andy Legg, who is 5ft 7in tall and weighs around 10 stone, can hurl a throw-in more than 46 yards.

SHORT THROWS

Long throws can put opponents under pressure, but in most circumstances a short and firm throw to a team-mate's feet is the best option. The priority is to retain possession from the throw. The responsibility for keeping possession does not only lie with the taker but also with his team-mates, who must make themselves available to receive the ball.

Players waiting to receive a throw should not stand rooted to the spot, for this makes it easy for their opponents to mark them and they thereby cut themselves off as potential outlets to the thrower. They should look for space and make their opponents think about their positions and intentions.

Players should keep moving and changing direction. They will lose their markers this way and, providing the thrower has read their intentions, they will be in a good position to receive the ball and retain possession for the team.

The thrower, too, when he has taken the throw, must get in a position to receive the ball. A popular and effective throw-in routine is for the taker to throw the ball and the receiver to lay it back into the thrower's feet.

A quick throw-in can also be useful, so a player should retrieve the ball quickly when it goes out of play, assess his options and make a swift decision about the possible advantage of a quick throw. In a defensive situation, a player may also be able to throw the ball back to the goalkeeper, who will be able to pick the ball up and kick it from hands. This is a useful option if the team is under pressure from the attacking team.

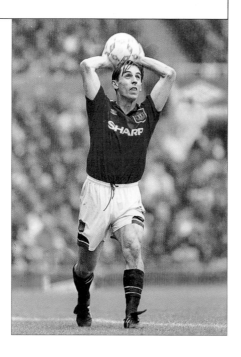

The long throw is an extremely effective attacking weapon. Here Gary Neville of Manchester United prepares to deliver the ball from touchline to penalty area.

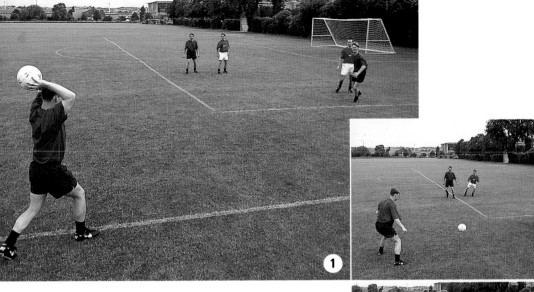

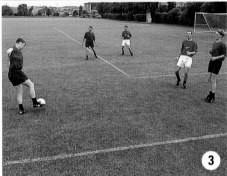

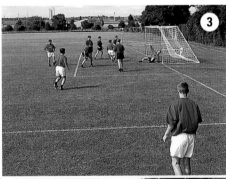

Like all set pieces, the first aim when taking a throw is to retain possession. If the defending team fail to mark the thrower, the following technique will ensure you keep the ball.
1. Team-mate drops of marker and comes toward thrower.
2. Throw is delivered to team-mate who returns the ball to the thrower.
3. The thrower now has the ball under control at his feet.

TAKING A THROW-IN

It is surprising just how many players get pulled up for 'foul throws'. So remember the basics:

- Always stand with both feet behind the touchline
- Keep both feet in contact with the ground at all times
- Take the ball right behind your head before releasing. This enables you to throw rather than push the ball
- Maintain your balance so your feet do not cross the line

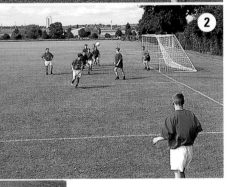

The long throw-in:
1. Try to deliver the throw hard and flat rather than looping the ball high.
2. At least one attacker should move to the near post to flick the ball on towards the far post.
3. The remaining attackers must time their runs to attack the ball as it is flicked on toward the far post.

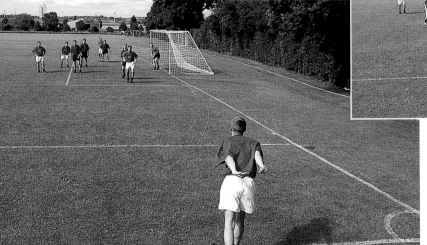

The biggest mistake players make when taking corner kicks is to just hit the ball into the penalty area and hope it finds a team-mate. That is not good enough and a waste of a good opportunity. Watch a decent player taking a corner and you will see that he has a plan in mind, a particular player he is trying to pick out.

corners

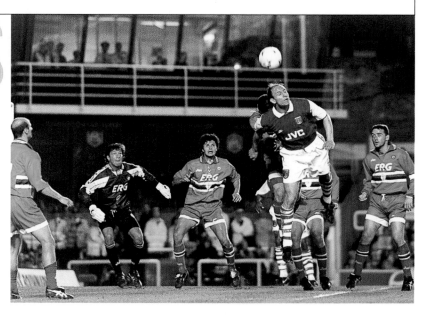

Arsenal defender Steve Bould gets up highest to flick on a near-post corner in the 1995 Cup Winners' Cup semi-final against Sampdoria.

CONSIDER YOUR OPTIONS

There are three main options open to a corner kicker:
1. the far post corner
2. the near post corner
3. the quickly taken corner

Whatever option you take, your priority should be to make the cross as difficult for the keeper to deal with as possible. A floated corner aimed towards the six-yard box, for example, is easy for any keeper to catch. If there is no real pace on the ball it will be no problem for the keeper to come and claim the cross. For the attacking side this is a total waste of a good situation.

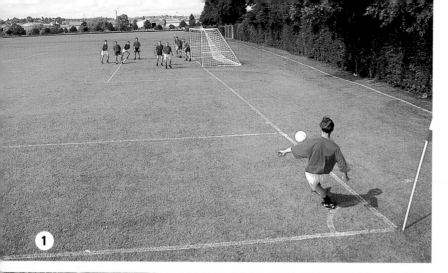

1

NEAR-POST

The near-post corner, in particular, is difficult for a keeper to deal with. He cannot reach it himself and has to rely on his team-mates to defend the situation. The ball should be delivered high to the near post and onto the head of an attacker. If the delivery is good, the ball will be flicked on by the attacker (though often a defender will inadvertently flick the ball on in an effort to clear the danger) into a dangerous area where team-mates will be trying to attack the ball and put it in the net. By the time the ball has been flicked on, the defenders are unsure where the ball is heading and the keeper is rooted to his line.

2

1. A good near-post corner must be driven in hard and not too high.

2. The player flicking the ball on must get in front of his marker and time his jump so the ball just flicks off his head.

3. Forwards attacking the flick must be positive in making their runs. They must also concentrate on keeping the ball down if they get a shot or header in on goal.

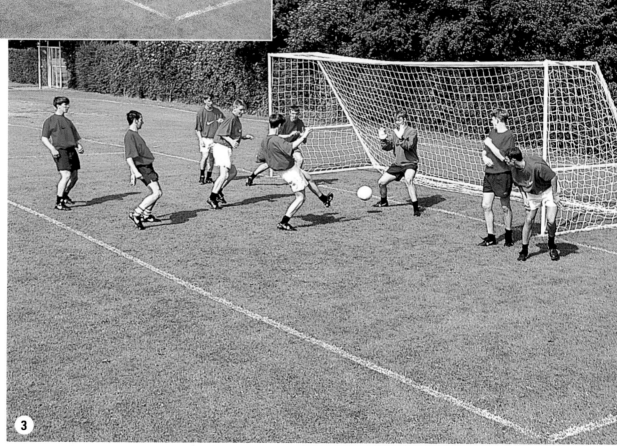

3

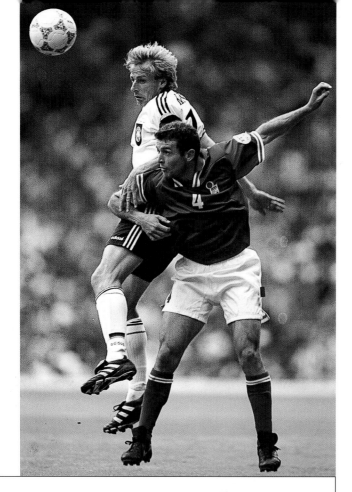

SHORT CORNER

If your options in the box are limited, the short corner should come into play. This is where an alert team-mate makes a run from the near post towards the corner flag, receives a little ball and returns it to the corner kicker who can deliver his cross (either high or low) from a different angle. By this time, attacking team-mates should have made their move and given the corner kicker the option of going for the near or far post.

The defenders will also have been pulled out of position and a decent cross could result in a goal. The only peril of the short corner is the risk of off-side. Defending teams can be quick to push out, so if you receive the ball from a short corner, don't be tempted to return it to the kicker if he is still in front of you...flags might be waved and an opportunity lost.

The near-post corner is fashionable, but the key to good corner-taking is to vary them so that the keeper is kept guessing. The short corner delivers the ball at a different angle and the far-post corner offers numerous options.

corners 2

Above: Jürgen Klinsmann beats his Italian marker to a corner in the 1996 European Championships. Even if you are unable to direct a header goalwards you should always challenge your marker and make it difficult for him to clear the danger.

TAKING A CORNER

A poorly delivered corner is frustrating for everyone, so make sure you take your time and hit a quality ball
- Time your delivery so that it coincides with the runs of team-mates
- Strike the ball with pace to make it hard to defend against
- Carefully consider your options. If the opposition are strong in the air, play a short corner to work the ball into the box

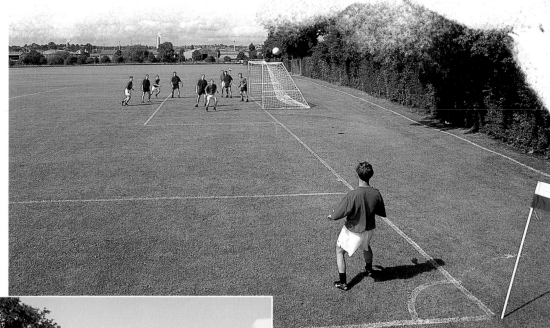

Far-post corners must be delivered with enough pace and height to elude the goalkeeper.

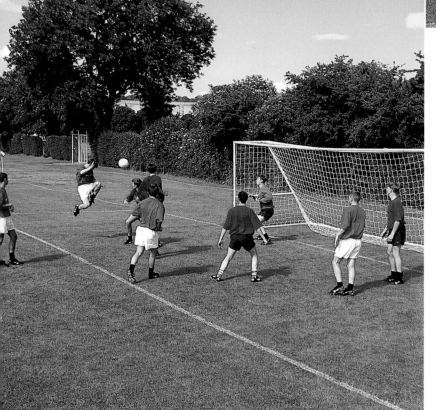

To win the ball from a far-post corner, attackers must drop off their markers and time their runs to arrive at precisely the right time.

FAR-POST

The far-post corner is a more straight forward option. A basic delivery, struck with pace to leave the keeper guessing as to whether he has time to come for it or not, is aimed for a team-mate at the back post. This is where the best headers of the ball should be positioned. Even if the ball is delivered properly, the attacker at the far post must still get enough power on the ball to beat the keeper. In most cases a left-footed player will take corners from the right (curling the ball in towards goal) and a right-footed player from the left. However this can make life easy for the keeper, so vary the delivery so that some swing in and some swing out and away from the keeper's reach.

A header from a far-post corner doesn't always produce a goal directly, but a header towards goal can cause chaos and confusion for the defence. But corners are not just about the kicker and 'the big guy in the middle'. Others on the attacking side play their part too. If you are taking a far-post corner, it is worth some of the smaller players making runs towards the near post as decoys. This will distract the defenders and keep them guessing. There's always a chance that some of these decoy players will be on hand to pick up the bits and pieces from any knock-downs.

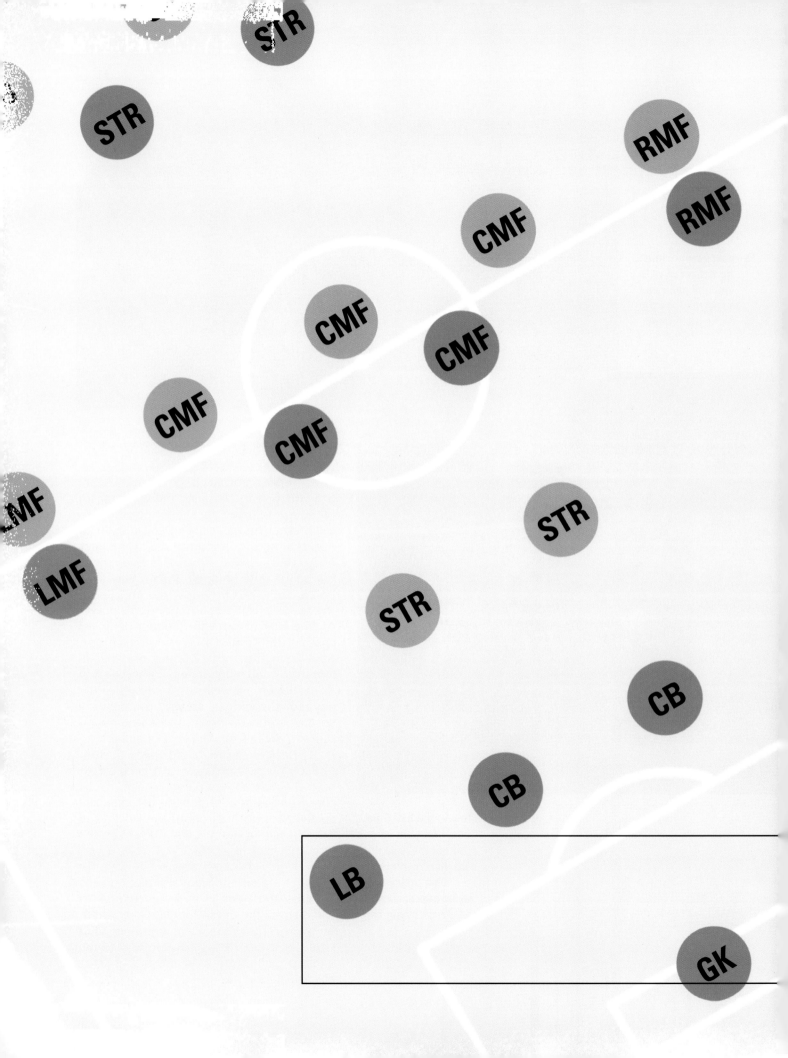

3
tactics

Players, rather than tactics, win matches. However, for players to fulfil their potential and play to the best of their abilities, they must have an appreciation of tactics and learn to play within different systems. The whole must be greater than the sum of its parts and the individual efforts of every player should complement the efforts of his team-mates. The German national team in the 1996 European Championship provides the perfect example of a team that worked to a system and outperformed more talented opponents. The variety of tactical systems available to coaches today is vast. Every league in every country seems to have a preference for a particular formation. When two systems clash, which regularly happens in European club football and international tournaments, coaches everywhere watch with interest to see which system fares better. In most cases, the quality of the players affects the result much more than the particular system being played, but it is still useful to discover the relative strengths and weaknesses of the different formations. The key to picking the right system is knowing who your best players are, what their strengths are and finding a formation that exploits their potential. Don't spend too long worrying about the opposition; concentrate on your own game.

tactics

In the modern game, strikers are expected to be versatile enough to play either alone in attack, or as one of a pair of forwards. Brazilian striker Ronaldo has to adapt to a different role when he plays for his club side, Barcelona, than that which he plays for his national team.

DEVELOPING GAME

The game of football is constantly evolving. Rule changes and greater fitness have made the game faster at all levels. As a result, tactics have had to evolve at a similarly furious pace. The back-pass rule, in particular, has affected tactics. Many teams now defend deeper and are unwilling to squeeze up to the halfway line as they used to. More teams play with a sweeper and this also presents coaches and managers with a problem because deep-lying defences are hard to break down. Putting the ball behind defenders and chasing it is no longer good enough. In many teams, midfield players have overcome this problem by developing the craft and guile to break down astute defences.

More and more teams are moving away from the traditional 4-4-2 formation and, instead, are using three central defenders – one invariably dropping back – and two wing-backs. Wing-backs are, essentially, fullbacks who have been given a licence to push on when their team is in possession. This is the single biggest tactical change we have seen in recent times. A similar change in attacking tactics has seen a new position behind an orthodox striker evolve. This position (often called the hole) is most famously occupied by Eric Cantona, Dejan Savicevic and Roberto Baggio.

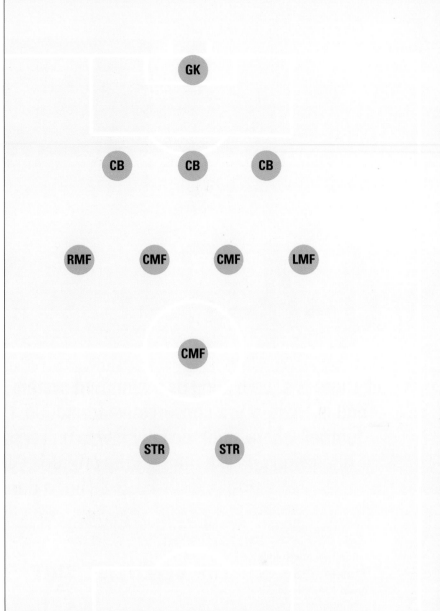

Above: 3-4-1-2 formations are increasingly popular in the modern game. They can be either attacking or defensive – largely depending on the role of the wide midfielders.

Left: AC Milan's Dejan Savicevic weaves his way through the Barcelona defence in the 1994 European Cup final. Savicevic is one of a number of modern forwards who occupies the position between strikers and midfielders. This position is particularly hard to defend against.

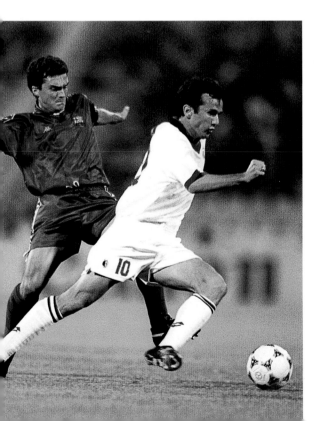

SYSTEM BY SYSTEM

In the next few pages, we will outline the most popular football formations. Many systems are subtle variations of others, and though we have not covered every permutation, we have outlined the most effective ways to switch your pattern of play during a game.

4-4-2

If there is such a thing as a 'standard system', it's 4-4-2. It uses only two forwards and is, therefore, a conservative formation. This system is very popular in British football where, until recently, it was universally employed at club level. Coaches and managers like the security offered by four midfielders and four defenders, but it does not have to be a negative system.

Spanish midfielder Fernando Hierra is a great example of the type of hard working midfielder needed in a 4-2-4 formation. In this system midfielders are often outnumbered and must be particularly industrious to make up for their lack of numbers.

THE DEFENSIVE UNIT

The foundation of a good 4-4-2 formation is defence. The back four (sometimes described as a flat back four) is made up of two centre-backs and two full-backs. The centre-backs are traditionally strong in the air as they must guard the penalty box from any threatening high balls. The centre-back pairing must develop a good understanding as they do not have the security of a sweeper operating behind them. The two players must decide whether to mark zonally, i.e. confine themselves to covering specific areas, or man-for-man, i.e. each take a striker and follow him for the whole game. A real threat to both marking practices, is the striker who drops back into the midfield to pick up the ball. The marker must decide whether to follow him (and thereby leave his central defensive partner alone at the back) or to pass responsibility for marking over to the midfield (though this may leave the midfield outnumbered). The only solution in this situation is to ensure that all opponents are marked and that the team keeps talking on the pitch, so that all players are aware of their changing roles. If just one player fails to appreciate the change you are in trouble.

The two central defenders are flanked by two full-backs (a left-back and a right-back). The full-backs play an important attacking role, but should not both go forward at the same time. This would leave the two centre-backs exposed to a counter attack. If one of the full-backs pushes on into a forward position, the opposite full-back should tuck in to support the central defensive pairing and, effectively, give the team three men at the back. The raiding full-back is now supporting a midfield which boasts five players so the traditional 4-4-2 has become a more modern 3-5-2. From this example you can see how different tactics and formations can overlap depending on circumstances.

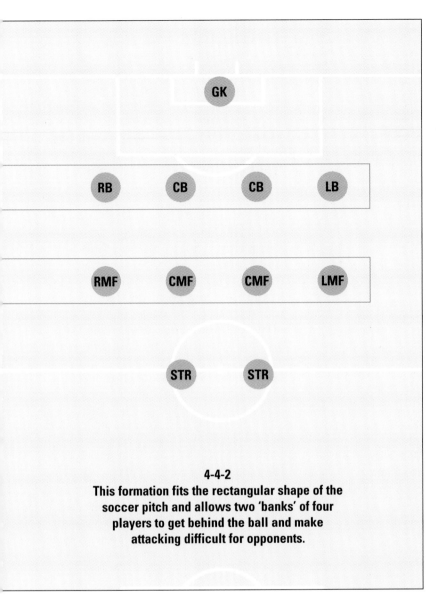

4-4-2

This formation fits the rectangular shape of the soccer pitch and allows two 'banks' of four players to get behind the ball and make attacking difficult for opponents.

THE MIDFIELD

The make-up of the midfield in 4-4-2 can be extremely varied. In the past, convention dictated that it should comprise, two wide-men (to patrol the flanks), a ball winner (to tackle and close down) and a play maker (to orchestrate attacking moves). Today, things are not so rigid. Some teams play with two ball players and two attacking wingers, while other teams employ two competitive ball-winners and two wide midfielders. Subtle changes in the midfield can turn an attacking formation into a defensive one.

4-4-2 INTO 4-2-4

A standard 4-4-2 system can quickly be converted to a more attacking 4-2-4 formation by simply pushing the two wide midfielders into a more advanced position, so that they operate as orthodox wingers. The 4-2-4 system is popular in its own right, but it does make great demands of the wide players. To be effective, it depends upon the wingers to get into attacking positions and deliver balls into the box for the strikers to feed upon. The option of playing the ball through the middle of the pitch becomes increasingly difficult, as the two central midfielders are likely to be outnumbered by their opponents.

AC Milan have been the standard bearers of 4-4-2 in Italy. Here Allesandro Costacurta stays tight on his man. With players of the quality of Maldini, Baresi and Costacurta in their defence, the flat back four has been extremely effective for Milan.

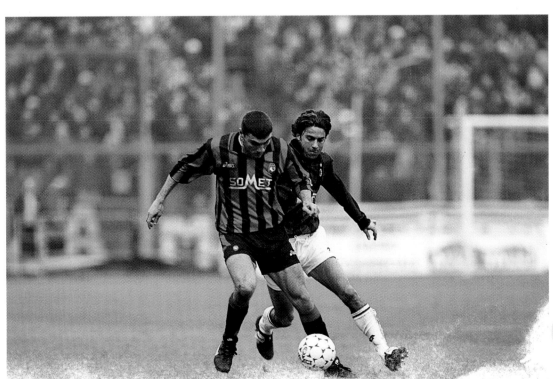

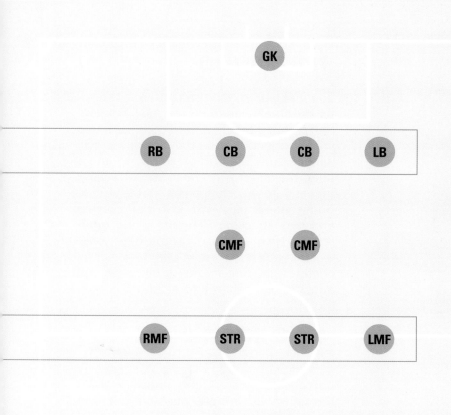

4-2-4
The more defensive 4-4-2 system can easily be transformed into a penetrating 4-2-4 system with wide midfield players pushing up level with the two strikers.

FORWARDS

The role of the two strikers in either 4-4-2 or 4-2-4 is very intensive. The pair must work together, both when in possession of the ball and when defending. The best strikers develop an understanding, so that, for instance, one makes a run to the near post and one to the far post, or one makes a decoy run while the other holds back for a square pass. Both strikers must work particularly hard when the ball is lost. With at least three defenders to pressurise, the importance of closing down effectively becomes paramount. There is no point in strikers charging around and diving at the feet of defenders; all it does is waste energy. Instead, strikers should close down (see page 98) and force an error. The days of the striker standing with his hands on hips waiting for a pass to feet are long gone.

ITALIAN IRONY

The flexibility of 4-4-2 has led to a number of Italian teams adopting this traditionally British system in recent years. Ironically, this has coincided with many English teams experimenting with the Italian-style sweeper system.

LEFT
The 4-4-2 system is the best platform for teaching players the importance of tactics. The four players at the back must work as a balanced unit, marking or closing down where necessary. For example, if opponents are attacking down the right, the defensive unit should work as follows:
1. Centre-backs must mark on the their opponents' outside, allowing them to intercept if the ball is played into feet.
2. The 'covering full-back' in this situation is the right-back (RB) and he must cover round the central defenders. But he must also be aware of the attacking position he has opened up (filled by the player marked LMF). He must be prepared to adjust his position accordingly.

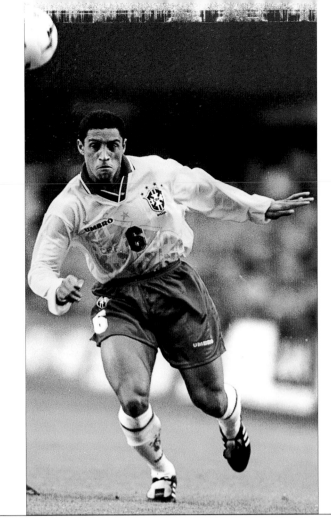

Attack minded full-backs like the Brazilian Roberto Carlos have easily adapted to the demands of the wing-back role. In many cases, it is the quality of the wide players which dictates the success or failure of the 5-3-2 system.

5-3-2

The current vogue in football tactics is for formations based on the 5-3-2 system. This approach gives coaches a degree of security with five defenders, but quickly adapts to an attacking 3-5-2 formation if needed.

3-5-2 OR 5-3-2

This type of system has been popular in most of Europe for more than 20 years, but when it was introduced into English football in the 1990s, there were murmurs of discontent and the suggestion the game would become too defensive. The general view was that the emphasis would be on preventing the opposition from scoring, rather than trying to score goals. However, this is not the case and like all systems 5-3-2 is as attacking as the players and coach want it to be. In many cases, teams are happy to attack from a solid base and with the use of wing-backs (full-backs with licence to get forward) a 5-3-2 formation quickly evolves into a 3-5-2 attacking option.

WING-BACKS

The role of the wing-backs is all important to this formation. They are the key to its success. To play in this position, you must be extremely fit (as fit as a traditional central midfielder) and you must have a full understanding of your responsibilities. You will be involved in all aspects of the game and must be proficient at attacking and defending.

You must support the midfield and front men when the team is in possession, but quickly revert to defensive duties when possession has been lost. It is a tough job, a demanding position in which to play. But when carried out correctly and successfully it can be one of the most rewarding positions on the field.

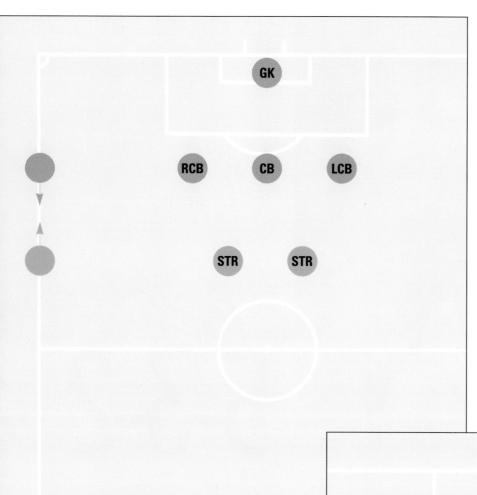

5-3-2 V 5-3-2

A game with two teams playing 5-3-2 can be negative. A stalemate can emerge as both teams fail to find gaps in crowded defences. This problem can occur when two teams play the same formation, whatever it is. What should happen, however, is that the team with the better players on the day wins the game. The team which wins the most one-on-one situations all over the park will come out on top in the end. Remember, tactics are only as good as the players who are attempting to carry them out.

(ABOVE AND LEFT)
The 3-5-2 system has become very popular in England over the last few seasons and is used by both Liverpool and Aston Villa. It relies upon three central defenders either playing in zones (above) or man-to-man marking with a sweeper (right).

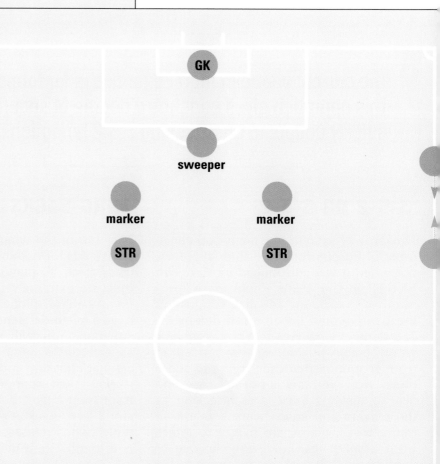

THE DIAMOND

Coaches and managers have tried variations on a familiar theme from time to time, and the diamond (4-1-2-1-2) system is one such alternative. Essentially, it involves a flat back four with one player sitting just in front of the defence; two central midfield players; a 'floating' attacking midfield player (or a striker operating in 'the hole') and two strikers. This system places a great deal of responsibility on the central midfield players to tuck-in and support the full-backs when they attack down the flanks.

4-4-2 V 3-5-2 (RIGHT)
By adopting this defensive shape (3-5-2), the red team can pack the midfield where they have five men against the blue team's four (who are playing a conventional 4-4-2 system) but still retain two out and out strikers.

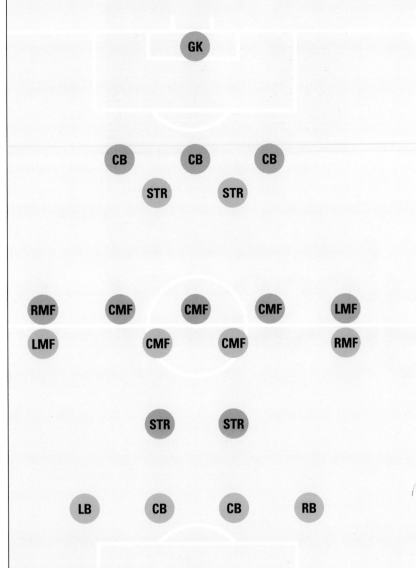

THE DIAMOND (LEFT)
This is a good system for a passing side, because both full-backs have space in which to attack. However, there are significant disadvantages against the more traditional 4-4-2 or 3-5-2 formations. The main problem is that, unless the two strikers get wide when their opponents have possession, the opposing full-backs will have time and space to build an attack.

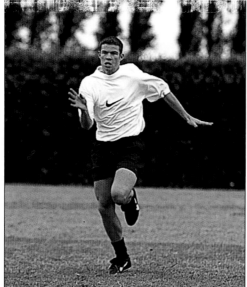

glossary

A

Aerobic training
The aim of aerobic training is to increase the flow of oxygen to the muscles. Endurance training such as swimming is an excellent example.

Anaerobic training
Exercise 'without air', (i.e. high intensity activity for example weight-lifting and sprinting). Anaerobic training can only be maintained for short spells.

B

Banana kick
Free-kick, often associated with Brazilian football. The ball is bent around the defensive wall and into the corner of the net.

Base fitness
The level of fitness which must be attained by players during the early stages of pre-season training.

C

Carbohydrates (complex)
Slow burning fuel for the human body. It's the most important part of an athlete's diet. Carbohydrate is stored in the liver and muscles as **glycogen** until being converted into glucose during exercise.

Good sources of complex carbohydrate include pasta, rice, bananas and cereals.

Carbohydrates (simple)
Fast burning fuel for the body. Simple carbs are commonly found in sugary food. They provide a short-term increase in energy level but do not provide any sustained gain. They should be taken to complement **complex carbohydrates**, not to replace them.

Closing down
Defensive technique used to deny opponents time and space.

D

The Diamond
A tactical system which employs four midfielders: one attacking midfielder to support the strikers; one defensive midfielder to take the ball from the defence; and two wide midfielders who 'tuck in' to protect the full-backs.

Diuretic
Substances which cause increased output of urine. Diuretics should never be consumed at half-time. Coffee, tea and alcohol are all diuretics.

F

Flat back four
A strategic formation, 4-4-2, in which the defence consists of two centre-backs and two full-backs who play in a line.

G

Glycogen
Sugar is stored in this form in the liver and muscles. Glycogen is converted to glucose during exercise and is burned in the muscle cells to produce energy.

H

High intensity training
Training intended to keep the heart rate at a level similar to that reached during a competitive match. This type of exercise should be complemented by sessions of **moderate and low intensity**, during which players work below their maximum capacity.

I

Isotonic drinks
Easily absorbed into the blood stream, an isotonic solution provides quick rehydration. A simple isotonic drink can be made by mixing fruit juice and water in equal measures.

L

Lactic tolerance
Lactic acid builds up in the muscles during activity as glucose is burnt in the muscle cells. A build up of lactate causes muscle pain. The length of time (and the extent of pain) which an athlete can endure and still continue to exercise is their lactate tolerance level.

Ligaments
Tough, fibrous tissues which link to the bone and reinforce the joint. Ligaments keep the joints in place while allowing great flexibility. Ligament injuries are common in football. It can take a great deal of time and rest for a ligament to regain its strength and flexibility once damaged.

P

Plymetric training
Training which develops explosive power within the muscles. Examples of plymetric training include jumping over hurdles and running across benches.

Power to weight ratio
This is an individual's muscle power as against their overall body weight. Muscle is very heavy and at a certain point it becomes inefficient (for footballers) to build and carry extra muscle.

Preparator
A qualified football trainer responsible for making sure that players are physically prepared to perform at their peak. Preparators are used extensively in Italy and are involved in training both with and without the ball.

Proteins
This is the main component of muscle and it is vital for growth. Protein takes a long time to digest and, contrary to pop-ular belief, is not a major source of energy. A healthy diet will consist of more **carbohydrate** than protein.

S

Sweeper
Defensive position which refers to the last player in a central-defensive trio. A sweeper usually plays alongside two markers and is responsible for patrolling the area behind his two colleagues. He is also expected to carry the ball out from the back.

T

Tendons
Tendons are linking agents which join muscles to bone.

The trap
The basic method of controlling a football using the foot.

W

Warm down
A short period of gentle exercise (similar to a **warm-up**) should be followed after every match. This will help breakdown any **lactate** which has built up in the muscles during exercise.

Warm-up
A warm-up should be carried out prior to any exercise. It is intended to raise the heart rate prior to competitive exertion and warm the muscles to make them more supple.

Wing-back
Variation on the full-back position. Wing-backs are usually used in a 3-5-2 or 5-3-2 system. They are responsible for patrolling the flanks and are expected to spend a great deal of the game attacking. However they must also defend their wing when required, as a result, this is a stamina sapping position.

Z

Zonal marking
Tactical system in which players are responsible for defending areas of the pitch rather than for marking particular players.

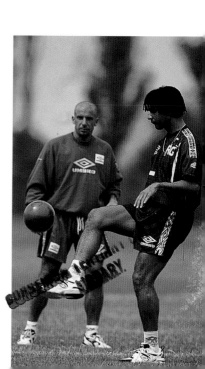

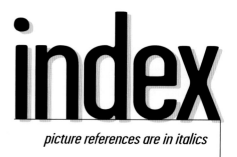

index

picture references are in italics

Free-kicks 100–103, *100*, *101*, *102*
Fruit 10, 11, 12, 13, 69

picture
acknowledgements

Allsport 4, 17 left, 22,
Shaun Botterill 76, 82, 84 top,
Simon Bruty 23,
Clive Brunskill 65 below, 86, 110,
David Cannon 94, 114,
Jonathon Daniel 92 top left,
Gary M. Prior 34, 68, 106,
Ross Kinnard 104,
Clive Mason 123,
Ben Radford 16, 78 top, 80, 88, 116, 119,
Mark Thompson 35, 96,
Claudio Villa 72, 90 left, 117
Colorsport 8, 12, 66, 69 below, 98, 100, 102 right, 102 left, 108,115,
Colorsport/Olympia/Martinuzzi 67,
Colorsport/Olympia/Ferrarini 69 top
Reed International Books Ltd 9 right
Richard Francis 1, 2, 5, 6, 17 right, 18 left, right, 19, 21 centre left, centre right, top right, bottom, 24, 25 top right, top left, bottom right, bottom left, bottom centre, 26, 27 centre left, top left, bottom right, bottom left, 28 right, left, 29 above centre left, above centre right, top, bottom, below centre, 30 top, bottom, 31, 32, 33 top, bottom, 36 left, centre, right, 37 right, left, 38 top, bottom, 39 centre right, top right, left, bottom right, 40 top centre, 40 top right, 40 bottom, 40 top left, 41 left, 41 right, 42 top, 42 bottom, 43 left, 43 right, 44, 45 top, 45 bottom, 45 centre, 46 right, 46 left, 46 centre left, 46 centre right, 47 right, 47 left, 48, 49 top, 49 centre, 49 bottom, 50 top left, 50 bottom right, 50 centre, 51 right, 51 left, 52, 53 right, 53 left, 54 top, 54 bottom, 54 /5, 55 right, 56, 57 right, 57 left, 58, 59, 60, 61 centre, 61 top, 62 below, 62 top, 63, 64 below centre, 64 below right, 64 below left, 65 top left, 65 top right, 70, 71 top, 71 below right, 71 below left, 74 , 75, 77 top right, 77 below, 77 centre right, 78 below, 79 top centre, 79 below right, 79 centre, 79 top right, 79 below left, 81 below centre, 81 top right, 81 below right, 81 top centre, 81 below left, 81 top left, 83 below, 83 top, 84 below centre, 84 below right, 84 below left, 85 top, 85 below, 87 below right, 87 top left, 87 below centre, 87 top centre, 87 below left, 87 top right, 89 below, 89 top, 89 centre, 90 right, 91 centre, 91 right, 91 left, 92 below right, 92 below centre, 93 below, 93 centre, 93 top, 95 centre, 95 below, 95 top, 97 left, 97 right, 97 centre, 99 centre right, 99 centre left, 99 top, 101 below, 101 top, 101 centre, 103 left, 103 right, 105 top centre, 105 top left, 105 bottom right, 105 bottom left, 105 bottom centre, 105 top right, 107 bottom right, 107 bottom left, 107 top left, 107 top right, 107 above centre right, 107 below centre right, 109 centre, 109 bottom, 109 top, 111 bottom, 111 top, 122, 179 top left,
David Jordan 11 centre,
Sue Jorgensen 11 top,
Jon Stewart 15
Clive Streeter 9 left, 13 top,
Philip Webb 11 bottom,
Trevor Wood 13 bottom
Hulton Getty Picture Collection 14
Roche Consumer Health 10

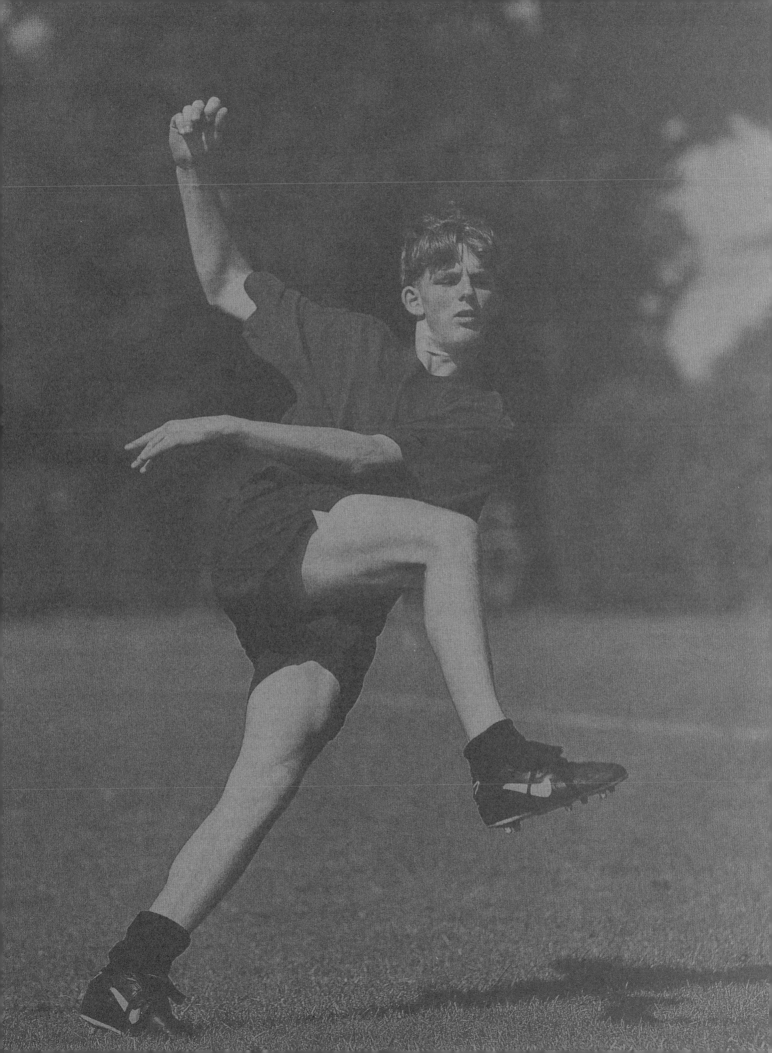

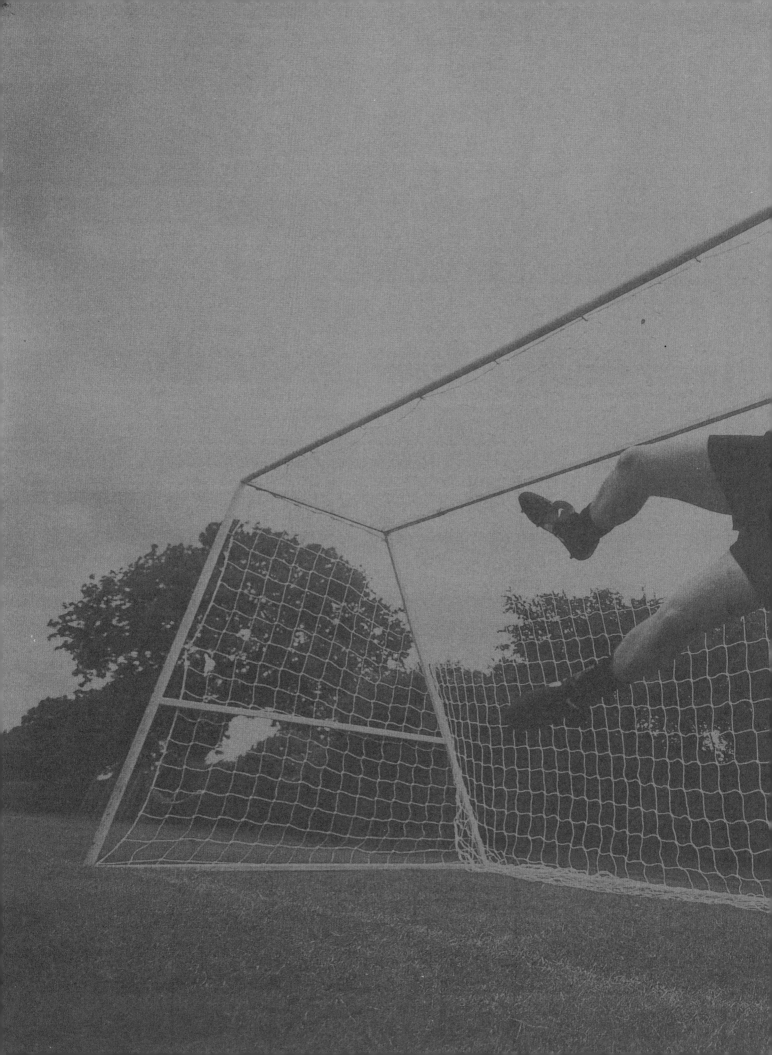